# Many Faces

by

# Terrie Starr

To my Spirit Sister
It's nice to Know that we
Can come back every few
years and ALWAys be the
same. I love you!
Jenni

I dedicate this book to the men in my life: My husband,
John, my "Starr in the East",
My sons David and Matthew, my shining stars
My grandson, David, my newest and brightest star
And, finally,
My dad, Sonny, my guiding star

# CONTENTS

# ACKNOWLEDGEMENTS

I want to thank all the people who, for over ten years have been so patient with me by reading every story at least a dozen times; every time I revised it; My sister, Gail, who has been my rock! My friend Lyn Coles, who convinced me when I was inconvincible, that I could write a book, that I should write a book; my friend, Jan, for always thinking that I am a better person than I do; Kymmy, whose enthusiasm and support have been incredible; to Kymmy's dad, George Rollin Parker III, who was such an inspiration in the writing of this book, and to Terry Ogden, my Parkinson twin, for the moving *Open Letter to Parkinson's disease*. And finally, my husband, John for his infinite patience and love.

# *4 AM*

4 AM is the darkest, loneliest hour of the day. Time stands still as
I ponder the same question as yesterday, the day before, and the
day before that-Is it morning or night?
There is no one to answer because I am the only person on the
planet awake.


4 AM is when I straddle the ditch that separates
morning from night.
Struggling in the heavy, opaque darkness to plant both feet firmly
On the morning side,
I stumble and trip over the air from my raspy breath as it
echoes through the house.


The silence is so loud that it hurts my ears.


4 AM is my daily wakeup call, my constant reminder, lest I forget
for one moment.
Parkinson's disease is alive and thriving within me.
It has awakened.

## WHO, ME?

Never before, in my life, have I considered myself a writer. I've been told often that I talk a lot or, more bluntly put, that I have a big mouth. Yes, I'm good at talking, but writing? I wasn't so sure about that when I received a phone call a few years ago. A nurse, Lyn Coles, had heard me speak at a health symposium in Indianapolis on Parkinson's disease. She called to tell me she thought I should write a book about my life experiences. "I don't know a thing about writing a book," I said, laughing.

"Just write like you talk. You have a story to tell," Lyn argued.

I wasn't so easily convinced. After numerous phone calls back and forth, and after Lyn promised to help me, only then did I agree to write my story. Well, folks, that was ten years ago, and I'm still writing it. Half of those years were spent trying to convince myself that I could write. The other half were spent in convincing myself that others would want to read what I'd written. So here it is: ten years worth of reflections of my thoughts and experiences through the first 53 years of my life. I hope that you will find something in my experiences that adds value to your life.

# BABY SISTER

No one detected her problems at birth. In the beginning, everyone thought it was just the normal delivery of a beautiful, healthy baby girl. She was born April 19, 1951. They named her Karen Lea. She was the largest of Mama's babies so far, weighing, at birth, a whopping ten pounds. Physically, they thought she was okay. It was not until her six-month checkup that her pediatrician, Dr. John Paul Jones, became alarmed. She was not developing as a normal six-month-old should. After extensive assessment, he delivered the devastating news to my parents. Mongoloid was the term used then. Down syndrome is the more appropriate diagnosis used today. Whatever name one chooses to use, they both mean the same thing.

Baby Sister, as she was very early on affectionately called, would never develop normally. Quite the opposite—as with most severely impaired Down syndrome babies, she was profoundly affected by this genetic disorder. Although, physically, she grew at a normal rate, in all other ways she would remain a baby. Mentally, she was severely and permanently impaired. She never crawled. She never talked. She never walked. She never lived to celebrate her 4th birthday. Compounding her mental limitations, she had congenital cataracts that rendered her virtually blind. She was deaf in one ear and had a hole in her heart—a hole that soon, would be left in the hearts of all who loved her.

Fortunately, Baby Sister was born into a strong, loving family—a family that loved and nurtured her throughout her short 3½ years. All those who knew her and those of us, like me, that knew only of her, were touched by her presence in their lives. Even the toughest and gruffest of men in the family, like

Uncle Oliver and Uncle Bill, were softened and made gentle in her presence.

I have seen only one picture of her. The image isn't clear enough for me to see her face, as she is cradled in Daddy's arms, wrapped in a blanket. If there were other pictures, they were gone by the time I was old enough to remember them. Gail, who was three when Baby Sister was born, has only vague memories of her. She remembers her crying. She does not remember her being called anything other than Baby Sister. I guess, in the memories of all who knew her, Karen was always a baby.

I never had the chance to know her. She died, at home, in Mama's arms, of congestive heart failure when I was 15 days old. Even though I never knew her, I do know that she was loved very much by all who knew her. One has only to see the look on Daddy's face in the picture as he gazes fondly down upon her.

# *LIFE WAS TOUGH*

Mama and Daddy's fourth child, I was born October 24, 1954 at a most inconvenient time. That's just my opinion, though. Think about the circumstances for a minute. Baby Sister died just fifteen days after I was born. She was really still just a baby, at 3½. Gail, the oldest, was six, and Mark was twenty months old. It's hard for me to believe that Mama and Daddy were just twenty-three and twenty-six at the time. We lived in a tiny house just a block from Hillcrest Heights Methodist church in Macon, Georgia. Mama was sixteen when she married Daddy. Just completing the 10th grade, she opted not to go back for her last year, the 11th grade, in those days. She had no marketable skills, and even if they could have afforded a car, she never learned to drive. She did what most women of the 1940s did: She stayed home and raised their children while Daddy worked the swing shift at a nearby Kaolin plant.

Daddy will be the first to admit that he was still just a boy when they became parents. Well, gosh, he was just nineteen when they married and twenty when he became a father. By the time I was born, he was twenty-six and still had not grown up. When he wasn't working, he was often out playing with the boys.

Mama didn't have the luxury of time out with the girls. She would often take all of us across town to see her mama, my Grandma Dorman. This was a major undertaking though. She was excessively fastidious about our appearance. She would have died a thousands deaths rather than have anyone see us barefoot with nothing on but a diaper. "Only common trash would let their child be seen in public with nothing on but a diaper," she'd say. Oh Lord, if we were old enough to walk, then we were too old to be wearing a diaper, let alone to drink from a bottle. She is very proud of the fact that she had Gail, Mark, and me potty-trained and weaned from the bottle at six months. Therefore, before we could go see Grandma, we all had to have a bath and put clean clothes on. Then, because we didn't own a car, we would all walk to the nearest bus stop, about three blocks away. Grandma lived on the south side of Macon, quite a few miles from our house. We would ride the bus to the end of the bus line and get off in the parking lot of an old car garage. From there, we still had a half-mile walk to Grandma's house.

My Uncle Oliver, Granddaddy Dorman's brother, worked in the garage and was always there to give me a wink, a bear hug, and a smile. Uncle Oliver was a confirmed bachelor, six years younger than Granddaddy. He lived right across the street from Grandma and Granddaddy in the old family home. I always fantasized that the real reason he never married was that he was secretly in love with Grandma.

Granddaddy and Uncle Oliver couldn't have been more different. Granddaddy, Earlie Dorman, was 6'7" tall, bald, lean, mean, self-centered, and abusive. By contrast, Uncle Oliver was 5'10", stocky, with a head full of red hair. He always had a smile on his face, a twinkle in his eye, and an old stogie hanging from the corner of his mouth. I was fascinated that he could talk without that old cigar falling out of his mouth. He was a sweet, loving, generous man.

Uncle Oliver was always there to watch over Grandma, Mama, Aunt Betty, Ronnie, and Ricky while they were growing up. Granddaddy would take off when the notion struck him and go on a big hunting trip. Often it would be at Christmas, and he'd leave Grandma without money for groceries or Christmas for the children. Uncle Oliver and one of Grandma's brothers, Uncle Jake, became the surrogate father that Granddaddy never was.

Uncle Oliver died on my sixteenth birthday, October 24, 1970. I can still see him clearly in my mind. With his weathered face, ruddy, and wrinkled from the sun, and those bright twinkling blue eyes, he had a look about him that made you think that he was either up to some kind of mischief or he had a secret that he was busting to tell. Although I was very young when Arthur Godfrey was a star, I thought Uncle Oliver resembled him. Mama laughed in surprise when I told her that. "He was a much nicer man than Arthur Godfrey was," she replied.

An old sea dog, Uncle Oliver, an ex-Navy man, was in the first battalion of SeaBees. Although his voice was gruff and gravelly sounding because of years of smoking, he had the gentleness of a lamb. His lap was always available to us to curl up in. I thought it was cool, as a little girl, to sneak a peek at the tattoo of the naked woman on his forearm. His was the first tattoo I had ever seen, a souvenir from his days at sea.

As children, we were never allowed to go inside his house. Not a very neat bachelor, he kept his mechanic tools and car parts on his living room floor. His "hootchy-kootchy" calendars hung on the wall in the kitchen. Even though he never married, he loved his women. On Saturday nights, he would go out "gal-ing." I suspect what the adults were afraid of was that we children would walk in on Uncle Oliver and one of his Saturday night "gals" and find them in a compromising position.

It was not until after his death, when we went in to clean his house, that we found, to our horror, the weight of all of those tools of his had caused the living room floor to cave in!

I like to think of Uncle Oliver as living quietly across the street, looking out for Grandma, Mama, and the other three, like a guardian angel. I think he was there, loving them all as his own and somehow as protection against Granddaddy's rage and abuse, and to make up for his selfishness.

# LIFE GOT TOUGHER

Mama had never experienced death before. She was only twenty-three when Baby Sister died. How could she have been expected to be experienced in the process of dying? Mama may have been naïve, but she was always a very intelligent and conscientious mother. She felt such guilt as though she, somehow, could have prevented Baby Sister's death.

How could she know that expulsion of bodily fluids was a natural process in death? She was embarrassed for anyone to see Baby Sister soiled. After calling Dr. Jones to tell him of Baby Sister's death, she quickly bathed and redressed her. Otherwise, she was afraid he would think she was a negligent mother.

It astounds me to think of all the responsibilities Mama carried on her young shoulders. In 1954, the year of my birth, Home Health services and Visiting Nurses were, as of yet, unheard of. Before she had a chance to recover from giving birth to me or to grieve over Baby Sister's death, one more burden was placed upon her. Daddy's mama, Grandma Willis, Lucile, was terminally ill with colon cancer at forty-nine. Daddy was an only child. His only sibling, Sydney, died of pneumonia at eighteen months. There was no one to care for Grandma while Granddaddy worked. There was no money to hire someone to care for her. There was no one to give her daily injections of morphine for pain. There was only Mama.

Mama loved Grandma Willis almost as much as she did her own mama. Daddy told me that when they heard the news of her cancer, he and Mama held each other and cried. Their hearts burdened, they cried for days.

It was logistically impossible for Mama to take care of Gail, Mark, me, and Grandma, too, living 30 miles away. The logical thing to do, which we did just weeks after Baby Sister's death, was to move from our tiny house in Macon to Grandma and Granddaddy Willis's house in Forsyth, Georgia. Mama cared for Grandma 24 hours a day for six months until her death in May 1955. I would expect that Mama was tired. I would say that she was emotionally spent, used up, if those were popular terms in 1955. Today she just says, "I did what had to be done. There wasn't time to think, let alone analyze my plight in life."

I spent most of my life, selfishly, wondering who could possibly have time for me. Who was there to rock me, hold me, sing to me, and give me the attention a six-month-old baby needed in order to thrive? There were so many needs of so many people.

I just recently found the answer to my lifelong question. A sixteen-year-old cousin, Margie Stowell, gave me the attention I needed. Margie's daddy, Uncle Buddy, and Grandma Willis were brother and sister. Grandma, Lucile, was the oldest in her family and Uncle Buddy was the baby. Their own mother had died when Buddy was two years old. Grandma, who was nine at the time, took on the role of surrogate mother to Buddy and the other children—Ollie, Agnes, and Millie—for several years until Papa Stowell remarried.

I guess, in a way, Margie was "passing it on." At sixteen, she looked around her family, searching for a place where she could be of help. She needed for someone to need her. She saw the burdens Mama was enduring. She asked Granddaddy's permission to move in with us to help. Margie was my answer. She is the one that changed my diaper, sang to me, played with me, and took me for walks. Thank you, Margie. I know now that I am who I am, partly because of you. Thank you for reminding me what a loving family we are.

# FOURTH PEW FROM THE BACK ON THE LEFT

Several years ago, while shopping in Macon, impulsively, my sister Gail and I decided to look for the church that we had attended when I was a baby. Hillcrest Heights Methodist Church was the name. I, personally, had no memories of attending this church. I knew only from family stories that this is the church we attended when Baby Sister died. We got lucky. Relying on Gail's memory from six years of age, we found the church. Unfortunately, it was locked and we were unable to find anyone to let us in.

Raised on Methodist doctrine, many of the rituals I have just taken for granted—Communion on the first Sunday of the month, the Apostle's Creed, singing the Gloria Patria, and responsive reading, just to name a few. There was one, though, that had always puzzled me. Why did we always sit in the fourth pew from the back on the left side of the church? It did not matter what church it was, we always sat in the same pew. Even, today, as an adult, I am not comfortable in a church unless I am sitting in the fourth pew from the back on the left side.

A number of years ago, I finally asked Mama why we had to sit in the same place wherever we happened to be worshipping. She responded, "Baby Sister died during the time our church was undergoing a big renovation. Your daddy and I bought a pew in her memory. There is a gold plaque on the end of the pew that reads, 'In memory of Karen Lea Willis, born April 19, 1951 and died November 8, 1954.' We paid $100.00 for that pew." That was a lot of money in 1954, a real sacrifice for Mama and Daddy. That pew was the fourth one from the back on the left side of the church.

One day, maybe I'll have a chance to find that church again and put my hand on the plaque and sit in our pew. Meanwhile, wherever I am, sitting in church in the fourth pew from the back on the left, I will always think about Baby Sister, the sister I never had the chance to know.

# AIN'T NO BUGGERS OUT TONIGHT

My first memories came at three years old, again, in Macon. We were living in a new sub-division called Sherwood Forest on Finsbury Drive. There was nothing particularly special about our house. I lived there with my older sister, Gail, and older brother, Mark, as well as Mama and Daddy. It looked much like the rest of the houses in the neighborhood—a three-bedroom concrete block house. The one special thing about the house was that it was ours! This was the second house Daddy had bought. He used his GI Bill to help finance the first one. The rest of the family thought we were rich because he was a homeowner at only twenty-seven. To buy a house at twenty-seven, even today, is not an easy feat to accomplish.

My memories begin here, rocking in the pink rocking chair, listening to Daddy sing. My lullabies were the top 40 hits of the 1940s: *My Blue Heaven, If I had a Nickel,* and *You Are my Sunshine.*

Still somewhat of a child himself, at least a child at heart, Daddy was our first playmate. Every day he would come home from work and teach us how to tumble, ride a bicycle, and how to catch a baseball. It is hard to say who had more fun.

In the days of my childhood, the late 1950s and early 60s, there was little to worry about concerning child safety; no drive by shootings, no carjacking, no gang revenge. In our little neighborhood, in Macon, we could wander all about visiting from house to house without the worry of us being kidnapped or molested—not that my parents would have had any ransom money anyway. If Mama needed me all she had to do was stick her head out the door and loudly call, "Yoo-hoo, Terrie, come home!" I was usually within shouting range because only rarely did we play inside someone's home. In addition, I wasn't allowed

13

to cross the street, so there wasn't very far for me to go. If the weather was nice enough to wander about the neighborhood, then it was probably nice enough to play outside. If I didn't hear her, a neighbor usually would. Whoever spotted me first would send me home.

These were the days before central cooling in the house or air conditioners in the cars. It was usually cooler to play outdoors. There was always a Crepe Myrtle tree or a Mimosa tree to shield us from the hot, southern sun as we played school or house or hide-and-go-seek. Ah, the thrill and anticipation of summer vacation! To me, it meant longer days, warmer nights, "playing out," swimming, and reading, and shelling peas, eating watermelon, and going to Grandma's house!

There was a certain mystique to playing outside at night. "Playing out" time called for different games, different rules, and different players: Tag, King of the Hill, Steal the Bacon, Red Rover, May I, Kick the Can, and last but not least, Ain't No Buggers out Tonight.

All the neighborhood kids would gather, just after supper, in the empty field across the street from my house—all the kids plus Daddy. He was always the "bugger." He had the loudest and deepest roar. One of his greatest thrills in life has always been to scare people. He was a bugger then. He's a bugger now. I'm sure he'd still like to play out at night if he could find anybody to play with him.

"Yoo-hoo, Gail, Mark, Terrie, Sonny, time to come home!"

# CALAMITY JANE

Calamity Jane was my nickname, and accidents were my bane. I have clocked more hours in the emergency room than many doctors have. Before I can even remember, I was making the ER run with Mama and Daddy for stitches. I was about eighteen months old when I had my first accident. We were living in Forsyth, Georgia with Granddaddy Willis. His house had a high front porch, about 15 steps up from the ground. There was a metal bar around the porch but nothing that would be child proof, better yet, Terrie proof. Therefore, I fell off the porch and landed right in the middle of a Pyracantha bush. Now, they are prickly enough by themselves, but this particular Pyracantha bush had a broken soda bottle in the center of it. Naturally, in addition to the scratches I received from the bush itself, I also gashed my forehead on the broken bottle.

I was two when I had my second set of stitches, also on the head—the chin this time. I was standing up in the plastic and metal chair that went to our 50s era dinette set. My feet slipped out from under me, and I fell chin first on the metal edge of the table.

Not long after, maybe a year, came the third trip when I was three years old. It was a beautiful summer night at Grandma Dorman's house in Macon, Georgia. She and I were playing outside on the concrete back porch. I found a piece of rope on the porch and talked Grandma into tying my hands and feet together so that I could hop like a bunny rabbit. This bunny rabbit stumbled and pitched head first onto the edge of the concrete porch. You guessed it. Another head injury, another trip to the ER and another set of stitches on the other side of my forehead. I have been told many times in my life that I am hard

15

headed. I have visible proof now. I broke a large chunk of concrete off Grandma's porch when my head hit it. Granddaddy went back later and etched my name and the date next to it.

As a child, I was very clumsy. Nothing physical came easily to me. I did not learn how to roller skate until I was thirty years old. Thank you, Jean Dickey, for your patience with me. You were one hot skating mama! I was almost eight before I finally learned to ride a bike. Our poor dog, Boots, nearly had a nervous breakdown while I wobbled around the backyard. She would run along beside me hour after hour while I practiced. I am sure her maternal instincts kicked in as she was trying to protect me. She probably thought she could catch me when I fell.

I never could hop more than twice on a Pogo stick, can't skateboard, I'm a lousy skier, and would flat fail a drunk driving test if I had to walk a straight line on command (even without being drunk).

Many years went by, though, with no trips to the emergency room. The last and most significant trip was in 1982 after being in a car wreck, in which I sustained a concussion. At least I did not need stitches that time.

I was a great cheerleader, an average tennis player, an average runner and cyclist, and a damn good aerobic instructor. I started teaching aerobics in 1980, teaching half the women in the county over a ten-year period. This was my passion. I had finally found my calling... until an undefined demon forced me to give it up in 1990.

# IT'S ALL IN MY HEAD

What seemed to be such an innocent comment made by a casual friend on a very ordinary day would become, later, an important life-changing event for me. Nothing about my life would ever be the same again.

I am oddly grateful for my jogging friend's keen observation. Thinking back over the events of the morning, I realized that I could no longer go on pretending there was nothing wrong. I'd been caught now. It was time to face the music.

My friend Kathleen and I were out running on a beautiful autumn Saturday morning in 1984. Coming towards us was Bobby, a friend and fellow runner. "Hey Terrie, how are you doing? You're holding your arm like you have a cramp in your side." Looking down at the crooked position of my right arm, hugging my side, motionless, I replied, puzzled. "No, we just started out. I'm not even warmed up yet. I hadn't noticed it until now."

That statement wasn't entirely true. The fact is that I had been noticing subtle changes in my body. So subtle, that I was hesitant to even give voice to them, thinking instead that my imagination was working overtime. The last thing I wanted was to be labeled a hypochondriac. It was frustrating that these were subtle changes that I could see, mostly feel, yet no one else, until now, had noticed. The arm thing that Bobby noticed was not a new thing. It had been hanging limply by my side for about six months, moving only when I told it to. It was also not a new thing that my rhythm and timing while teaching aerobics was diminishing. Additionally, I was losing the fine motor coordination in my right hand. Because others hadn't noticed anything wrong, it was difficult to talk about it.

17

I had been married to a man, Dave, for ten years, and even he hadn't noticed anything wrong. Therefore, I would just try to push the thoughts out of my mind.

I returned to college at thirty years of age to finish a degree that I'd started at eighteen. After ten years of marriage, college was my salvation for the divorce I was going through at the time. It was also my way of fighting the inevitable passage of time.

Walking across the open spaces of Georgia College's beautiful campus in Milledgeville, Georgia became increasingly difficult. I could not seem to walk in a straight line; instead, I teetered off to one side or the other, dragging my right foot. Getting from point A to point B on campus became a struggle. Just to be certain I wasn't going nuts, I examined the shoes in my closet. For sure, the toe of every right shoe was scuffed, proof that, for some reason I was dragging my foot. Even when I concentrated, I couldn't pick it up more than a step or two. The time had come to give all my high-heeled shoes away. There was no way I could walk in them and maintain my balance.

At the time, I wasn't worried about life-long debilitating disorders. The symptoms, at the time, subtle, were just a minor irritant. No one else seemed to notice. That had its good side and bad side. The good side is that I wasn't drawing attention to myself; consequently, I worried that perhaps, I was just imagining them. I knew that I really should see a doctor, if for no other reason than to quit obsessing over it. I had been telling myself that for months. I had mixed feelings. I was scared to find out it could be some devastating disability and yet, I feared I would find out it was all in my head. Which would be worse, I wondered?

I continued going to class every day. I continued teaching aerobics four days a week. I continued to be a busy, active, single mom to David and Matthew, then seven and four. I continued to recover slowly and painfully from my unforeseen divorce from Dave. In addition, I continued to worry about these nagging symptoms.

Finally, I guess I worried about it so much that a good friend of mine, Greg Jarvie, who was my psychology professor at the time, asked me what was wrong. With his support, thus began a four-year journey to countless doctors, through numerous tests searching for what appeared to be a needle in a haystack. As the years progressed, the symptoms increased in number as well as intensity. Of course, the stress did, too.

I continued life as usual—go to school, care for David and Matthew, teach aerobics, study, enter the world of dating, worry about my increasingly worsening symptoms, and periodically go to different doctors only to hear them say, "I don't know."

In 1987, a momentous year for me, I graduated from Georgia College with a degree in Community Health; I bought my first new car, a 1987 red Dodge Daytona; started a new job, the first one in quite a few years, as a Social Worker. I moved David, Matthew, and myself to Milledgeville, Georgia; and I found a doctor at Emory University in Atlanta that told me something other than, "I don't know."

He said two words to me that had never been said to me nor had ever occurred to me: Parkinson's disease. I was stunned. I didn't know whether to be relieved that I wasn't crazy or depressed that I'd just been given a diagnosis of an incurable, chronic, progressive neurological disease. There must be some mistake. Parkinson's disease is a disease for the elderly, isn't it? I was just thirty-two!

Initially, I was relieved that I wasn't crazy. There was no way, in the early years of the disease that I could even imagine the full extent of the impact this would have on every minute of every day for the rest of my life. I think a better way of describing the way I handled the diagnosis would be to say I was in denial. On some level, I was cognizant to the fact that not only was it NOT going away but that it would get progressively worse. Denial was a wonderful coping mechanism at the time though. I was too young to be able to comprehend what I would have to endure over the years to come. How could I truly comprehend something I had never seen before? If I knew then what I know now, I'm not sure I would have survived.

It's been twenty-five years since this life began. Living with Parkinson's disease has been somewhat like going to battle with the devil. Sometimes, I take my medication and I can be in control. Sometimes, no matter what I try to do, Parkinson's disease is in control.

*A dear friend of mine, Terry Ogden, whom I would meet a few years later, wrote a very moving* Open Letter to Parkinson's disease. *It so accurately describes how Parkinson's disease has affected my life, his own life, and I'm sure, the lives of countless others.*

## *AN OPEN LETTER TO PARKINSON'S DISEASE*
### By
### Terry Ogden
### 2/12/95

I know you.
It took some time and a lot of pain,
Now I know you and what you are and what you do.
And tragically—how you do it.
I hate you.
I say this without rage and not out of an emotional fever.
I say it coldly, logically and with all my faculties in tact.
I hate you and as long as I draw breath, you are my mortal enemy.

You came into my life unwelcome and uninvited.
You began as an inconvenience; a nuisance.
And I adjusted and went on, but you weren't satisfied.
A shaking hand, an unsteady grip, a stiffening gait was just your introduction.
You eventually robbed me of the pleasure to be found in the simple act of a casual stroll, or writing a letter, or taking a drive.
Still I tried to adjust, abide and endure.
But the irritation became an obstacle and the obstacle became a torment.
What had begun as a physical encumbrance, all too soon became a way of life.
Ever-present, all encompassing, affecting every moment of every day.

And at the end of each day, you deprived me of the sleep that might have given me strength to face the next.

I am not alone in my struggle.
I have wonderful friends who understand all that they can and forbear what they cannot.
I have a loving and constantly supportive family, who amaze me with an unending well of compassion, patience and stamina.
And I have a life partner who is my lover, my best friend, my strength and now my partner in pain, because she must bear my suffering, but without the refuge she gives me.

The passion with which I love my family is infinite and unbounded.
It never diminishes and grows with each passing hour.
And, in kind, because you seek to injure and torment my family,
With this same unbounded and infinite passion do I hate you.
What you have done to me would be more than enough to deserve my hatred.
But, you see, all you do to me, in turn, hurts those I love.
And that I cannot tolerate.

What did you take from me?
If I might overlook the loss of productivity and recreation,
If I could forget the physical pain and the endless hours wasted in repeated attempts to accomplish the simplest of tasks. There is another assault that I cannot ignore.
In the taking of my simple dignities you have depleted my tolerance.
In taking away my power and clarity of speech, you rob me of my need to communicate, to express myself, to teach and to learn.
When you block my ability to dress myself, feed myself and to provide for myself the basic needs of each day you steal from me the absolute primal human need for dignity and an embraceable self-image.

That's when I saw you for what you truly are.
After turning me into a physical caricature of the person I once was,
After taking away my mobility, productivity and creative abilities,

22

After altering the very nature of how I led my life, you assaulted the last remaining vestige of the quality of my life; my simple human dignity.

That's when I knew you for what you are.

You are a bully and indeed, all bullies are cowards.

When I recognized you for the cowardly son of a bitch that you are,

That's when I gave myself permission to hate you.

Hate can be destructive and counter-productive and as such should usually be avoided. But when we encounter evil, injustice and cruelty, we are entitled to hate with an unbridled self-righteousness.

If ever evil existed, it is you.


I now know how to fight you.

You glory in what I cannot do, in what you can deprive me of.

So, I will fight you with all the can-dos in my arsenal.

If I get out of bed, you lose.

If I get dressed, you lose.

If I can produce, create, nurture, learn, grow or be of help to anyone, anywhere, you lose.

It is a battle of one hour at a time and each hour brings me the chance to look you in the eye and say with all the voice I can muster "I DO NOT FEAR YOU".


I know you now for a coward and a bully and I know that as such, you thrive and grow on fear, despair and hopelessness.

But this is where your power ends and mine begins.

My courage and hope can only be taken by you if I give them to you.

I control these and as long as I live, they will be steadfast and ever strengthening,

Because I know how badly you desire this last bastion of my sanity and self-worth.

Hope and courage, these are my weapons and with them I plan to beat you to a whimpering and cowardly submission.


It is only fair to warn you that in my fight, there are many soldiers; scientists, doctors, surgeons; who at this very moment are planning and progressing towards your ultimate and irrevocable demise; caregivers, who, though not afflicted themselves, live with the suffering through their love and stand shoulder to shoulder with their loved ones to hasten your defeat. And across the world, millions of my brothers and sisters you have victimized, tormented and abused.

We all hate you.

We will not fear you.

We defy you.

You cannot last.

You will lose.

Now it's time for you to be afraid.

# NEW RELATIONSHIPS

September of 1987 marked the beginning of two lifelong relationships. The first relationship formed was with a world-renowned expert on Parkinson's disease, Dr. Ray Watts, a man who over the years would become as much a friend and colleague as my personal doctor. The second lifelong relationship was with the medication necessary for me to be a functional human being.

There were years of trying to wait patiently through the agonizingly slow approval of new drugs by the FDA. Once the FDA finally approved the drug, there was the daily battle of trying to introduce the new drug to my system, praying that I could tolerate it without horrendous side effects. There were always side effects to endure—the good, the bad, and the ugly—but also the excitement that maybe it will be this drug that will restore my functional level back to normal. Maybe this drug will be the cure I have been praying for.

There was always nausea as my system adjusted to the latest "poison." The dilemma: do I take it on a full stomach or an empty stomach? I will never forget those mornings of hugging the base of the commode in the bathroom of my office as I vomited repeatedly, praying for the day the newness of the drug would wear off, and I could feel human again. Finally, the resignation that this drug wouldn't be the cure I'd prayed for either. I still had Parkinson's disease, and I would have it next week, next month, and next year. All of the new drugs, thus far, have been a temporary fix. When the drugs wear off, I still have Parkinson's disease.

Meanwhile I had a life outside of Parkinson's disease. I just had to figure out how to make my life and Parkinson's disease work together. That was not an easy task. I'm very blessed to have been born with a great sense of humor. It pulled me through some rough periods in my life. Humor also helped my sons, David and Matthew, to keep it all in perspective. Parkinson's disease was simply a part of our lives, a part that we all tried not to give too much attention to. I found out early on that the more attention I gave to the disease, the more attention it demanded. We all had far too much living to do to let a neurological disorder compromise our lives. Of course, my children were forced to live with it, too. They didn't have the luxury of denying its existence any more than I did.

I don't know when, if ever, they have thought of me as being handicapped. In fact, I didn't see myself as handicapped either. Part of the denial game was not to look into too many mirrors. That way I never saw myself as others did.

It was in 1990, I think, when I finally admitted to myself that my life would be just a little bit easier if I had a handicap tag for my car. It may have looked a little odd to see a 30 plus - year-old mom driving a red Daytona with two kids, a dog, a drum set and a handicapped license tag on the rear of my car. David and Matthew thought it was very cool to park in the reserved spaces at the shopping malls. They had their own name for the handicap tag. They called it "Mom's retard tag". I'd rather have a warped sense of humor than no sense of humor.

When David and Matthew were young, they had a set of toy people called *Weeble Wobbles*. They were brightly colored, egg-shaped people. You could knock them over, but they would pop right back up again, never really falling down. One of David and Matthew's favorite games to play with me was the human version of *Weeble Wobble*. Guess who the *Weeble Wobble* was? Matthew would position himself on one side of me and David on the opposite side. They would push me back and forth from one to the other. One particularly bothersome symptom of Parkinson's disease is impaired balance. Merely to push me lightly with a finger would send me falling. Careful not to actually let me fall, the boys would push me from side to side, catching me just *before* I fell, and then they would push me back the other way. They thought it was funny to have a *Weeble Wobble* Mom. I thought it was cool to have sons with such a good sense of humor.

One night, around the same period, friends of David's were at our house talking about how tough and strong they were as fourteen and fifteen years old. They were strutting around flexing their muscles and generally acting like macho men. Amused, I challenged each of them to test their strength by Indian leg wrestling me. There was considerable grinning and winking, each thinking they would be wrestling a wimpy woman. Clay Harrison, the most physically fit of them all said, "Are you sure, Miss Terrie? I don't want to hurt you."

"Get on the floor, Clay," I said, winking at the other guys. Clay looked at David, Brian, and Ed in bewilderment as though to ask, "What did I do?" After locking arms, hips lined up evenly, we began the leg lifts as we counted; one, two, three, lock legs and flip! Clay slowly rolled out of the backward flip I put on him while his cheering section was shouting, "Man! Wow! I don't believe it!"

Looking at the stunned expressions on their faces I calmly asked, "Next?"

# *Now What Do I Do?*

The harsh reality that Parkinson's disease was in my life to stay became clear to me on April 20, 1992. I retired this day from a career that I loved very much. I had been a Medical Social Worker since graduating from college in 1987 at the age of thirty-two.

I started my career as a Case Manager, visiting with and helping the elderly manage their health care needs at home. Two years later, the Administrator of a nearby hospital asked me to be the Director of Social Services at a county hospital thirty miles from Sandersville, Georgia, where I lived in the rural, central part of the state. I accepted the position and as much as I loved that job, after two years, I could no longer afford, physically, to subject myself to the high stress level and the constant acuteness that the job required. My Parkinson's symptoms exacerbated dramatically in the two years I worked there. I still needed to work for financial reasons, but I really needed to scale down the demands of my job for the sake of stress. I negotiated a contract with a local nursing home to provide social services and activities for the residents of the center. I managed to work through a year's contract. When my contract came up for annual renewal, I was simply "out of gas." The physical toll, just the effort of going to work every day and trying to meet the challenges that my job brought, was making me worse fast. April 20, 1992, I sat in the office of Social Security Administration for my face-to-face interview with a social security representative to begin the process for determining my eligibility for disability. There are no words to describe how it felt to be thirty-eight years old, with two children, a dog, a house payment, a car payment, insurance, medication, and a boyfriend, facing the reality that I could no longer physically hold down a job. How could I even imagine maintaining a relationship?

Here is where I think our Social Security program fails us. To apply for disability, one must prove unemployment upon submitting the disability application. The determination of eligibility process takes six months. For me, that meant six months of no income. There is no allowance in their system for gradually scaling back on the amount and frequency one works. It is all or nothing. I was one of the lucky ones. I have a sister and father that took care of me financially until social security made its determination. What I want to know is what happens to the people that are not fortunate enough to have family with the financial means to support them through the six-month waiting period? Moreover, what happens to those people to whom social security denies disability eligibility?

Exactly six months after my initial interview, October 20, 1992, I received my official social security stamp of approval for total and permanent disability. This was to be my 38th birthday present. Now, what would I do with the rest of my life? The next twelve months proved to be the worst year of my life as I struggled to hang on to a failing, destructive, romantic relationship and strived to adjust to my newfound position in life. My symptoms increased. The side effects of the very medication I had to take in order to be a functional human being were causing side effects as debilitating as the disease. The medical term for the side effect is dyskinesia. It means excessive, uncontrollable movement. Here was my dilemma: I could stop taking my medication, and then I would not be able to move, walk, or talk clearly. On the other hand, I could take the medication and live with wild, uncontrollable movements, a flailing and jerking of the right arm and leg. I chose the latter. This meant, though, that I would constantly call attention to myself, as I moved about with no control.

Attention is not what I wanted. I'd have been happy to be invisible. This is why Parkinson's disease is known as the invisible disease in the young onset group. One would expect an elderly person to have Parkinson's disease but certainly not a young person like me! People watched me, though, and formed their own opinions about me. I don't know why that bothered me as much as it did.

Rumors were flying around my small southern town. She's drunk! She's on drugs! She's crazy as hell! Dyskinesia interfered with every aspect of my life. It overrode anything else I tried to do at the time. Even to carry on a conversation was difficult. Trying to engage in a telephone conversation and hold the telephone to my ear at the same time was nearly impossible. Holding the telephone with an uncontrollably flailing arm while simultaneously trying to listen and in turn speak; that is, to formulate the words in my brain and somehow get them out of my mouth in a coherent, fluid fashion became a complex process. It is a process, like many others, that we take for granted until something happens to break the flow of task, thought, and movement.

As conspicuous as I was to others when dyskinetic, though, I always preferred that to the frozen, statue-like "off" state. Most of my friends with Parkinson's disease would agree with me. Oddly enough, I felt more comfortable and more in control when dyskinetic. I was not realistically aware of how noticeable the dyskinesia was to others. It was not until a couple of years later, while viewing a television interview of me, that I saw myself through the eyes of others. It looked even worse than I thought!

By the spring of 1993, I was profoundly depressed and severely impaired. I didn't want to leave the privacy of my home. I hated the fact that the erratic, uncontrollable symptoms constantly called attention to me. I felt like I was banished to the sidelines of life, sitting on the edge, watching others participate in a life that I no longer felt a part of. Why me, God? If I was now questioning God, I could no longer depend on denial to shield me from the harsh reality of this damned disease. Surely, I could not spend the rest of my life like this.

There had to be a reason for this hell I was living in. Why me?

# THE REASON

Emory University in Atlanta is a wonderful place to go if you have anything seriously wrong with you. I have thanked my lucky stars, my insurance coverage, my family, my doctors, and God every day for the past twenty years for the good fortune of having some of the best neurologists in the world taking care of me. Out of the million plus Parkinson's patients in this country, alone, only about 10–20% fall within the group known as, "Young Onset Parkinson's disease." Dr. Watts, a noted specialist in movement disorder, would naturally have reason to see more patients in this sub-population, such as me, than other less specialized neurologists. I was somewhat a novelty, even to him, though, let alone the rest of the team of doctors that I would come to know well enough to call them my family.

I think I was a novelty for several reasons. I could date my symptoms back at least to 28 years of age. Since 80% of all dopamine-producing cells are dead by the time the symptoms of the disease appear, that means I had had the disease for much longer than that. At the time I first met Dr. Watts, few patients in my age bracket were being diagnosed, probably for the same reason it took four years for my own diagnosis—doctors didn't know to look for it in someone as young as I was.

As I have stated, I have what is called Young Onset idiopathic Parkinson's disease. Idiopathic means simply that the cause of the disease is unknown. Because I was very young, I had no other medical problems to get in the way and mask the symptoms that Parkinson's disease presented. For someone trained to diagnose Parkinson's disease, despite my age, the disease was very clear cut and easy to see.

The disease progressed in me very rapidly to the point that I was severely impaired and was experiencing dramatic side effects to the drugs very early on. Much like going from zero to 100 mph in five seconds, Parkinson's disease went from subtle to severe in five years.

Depression had become a huge factor by the time I saw Dr. Watts in Feb. 1993 for my six-month check-up. I guess you could say that I was profoundly depressed. I did not want to kill myself—I wanted to LIVE, but I was no longer able to live my life with the quality of life that was acceptable to me. I was willing to try anything for a chance to restore some semblance to a life that I once knew.

Dr. Watts gave me a ray of hope not long after that February appointment. He referred me to a surgical team of neurologists and a neurosurgeon who were involved in a study of surgical intervention in Parkinson's disease. The procedure - Microelectrode Guided Pallidotomy, and they were following 15 successful outcomes. If I passed the extensive pre-operative screening process, then I would be their 17th patient as well as their youngest to date.

I will never forget a conversation I had with Dr. Vitek just prior to my procedure. We were sitting in his small office in Emory's neurology research center. Casually, he asked me what I most wanted to do after the surgery that I could not do at that time. Without hesitation, I said, "I want to play tennis with my Dad" (who was recovering from quadruple bypass surgery a month earlier). Dr. Vitek had a very concerned look on his face and slowly shook his head. "Oh no, Terrie! I'm afraid you are being unrealistically optimistic." I smiled, "Just wait. You'll see."

It was my chance of a lifetime, and I hung every hope I had ever had on the outcome of that procedure. I had the support of my family, my children, my friends, and my entire town. People that I didn't know at churches I had never been to were praying for me. Several months of trips to and from Emory, prior to my surgery date, all pre-op testing was completed satisfactory, and I was sitting on ready, willing, and determined to make the most of this opportunity given to me. I knew just how fortunate I was when I found out, immediately after my surgery, because of my well-publicized success, that the waiting list had grown to three years! I'm getting ahead of myself though.

Pallidotomies were a reintroduction of an old surgical technique with a new twist—the Microelectrode guided brain mapping. Emory was on the cutting edge of a huge scientific breakthrough, and the public relations department wanted to tell the world. Dr. DeLong, then head of Emory's neurology department, wanted to be very careful which patient he featured for the story that CNN would tell the world. In short, he picked me to be the patient that would tell their amazing story.

It surprises people when I tell them that I had no fear leading up to the surgery. None whatsoever! Something deep down in my soul told me that there was no reason to be afraid. I knew the outcome would be what I wanted. Besides, I had all the confidence in the world in my team of doctors. I had come to know them all intimately over the months we'd been together. They were like family to me. In addition, I had spent the past year or more questioning why I was cursed with such a visible, debilitating disease. I always felt there had to be a reason for it. Never did I think it was something God had given to me as punishment for some terrible sin I had committed. Little did I know that I was very soon to find the answer to my question, "why me?" Dr. DeLong picked me to be the person to give hope to the hundreds of thousands of people with Parkinson's disease. CNN covered my story from before my surgery, through the surgery itself, and would follow my recovery for more than a year.

October 27, 1993, the day of reckoning, had come. At 6:00 AM I had my army of supporters in my hospital room when the neurosurgical resident came to start the day by putting my halo on. I am not going to lie. That was the most painful part of the entire day, and the only time during the entire procedure that I wanted to wimp out. My friend, Greg Jarvie, was part of the support group congregated in my hospital room. When the surgical resident gave the order for everyone to clear out of the room, I grabbed Greg by the hand and said, "Greg stays!" One of his specialties is in pain management.

Greg sat in front of me, holding my hands, and helped me focus on anything other than the pain. How do I describe the pain I experienced having the halo put on my head? Imagine what it would feel like to have your head clamped inside a vise and have someone turn the handle on the vise as it gripped your head tighter and tighter until it feels like the skull bones are going to snap.

Once the halo was on and final pre-op tests done, the resident took me straight to the operating room. Operating Room #15 was the standard Pallidotomy operating room. It was very cold, quite small, and very crowded. I think I counted fifteen people in there at one time, most of them hovering under warm blankets, shivering from the low, refrigerator-like temperature of the room.

Two of the three key players on the Pallidotomy team greeted me immediately—Dr. Mahlon DeLong and Dr. Jerrold Vitek. Dr. DeLong, Chairman of Emory's Neurology Department, reminded me of a cross between Star Trek's Mr. Spock and an absentminded professor. Soft spoken, devoid of accent, he had a quiet, thoughtful, and calming presence about him. He was in his mid-fifties at the time, I would guess. Tall and slim, he was bald and had vibrant blue eyes hiding behind wire-rimmed glasses. He always gave me the impression that he had just misplaced something very important. (The funny thing is, usually, he has!) His appearance of absent-mindedness masked his incredible intelligence and dry wit.

Dr. Vitek, Jerry, with a boyish appearance, looked much younger than his years. He was two years older than I was but looks, easily, ten years younger. When I think of him, he reminds me of the little boy on the Wheaties commercial, dressed up in an oversized basketball uniform. Born and raised in Minnesota, his accent was quite distinct. But one should not allow his youthfulness to belie his skill and knowledge. He has a special gift of translating the most technical medical terminology into a language that most anyone could understand. Polite and respectful, he had a wonderful bedside manner. He always treated his patients and their families as though they were friends.

I remember looking at the clock as soon as the nurses transferred me to the operating table. It was 10:00 A.M. when Dr. Bakay, the neurosurgeon, locked my halo down to the head of the operating table and began shaving my head and prepping me for the initial burr hole in the top of my head with what sounded very much like an ordinary drill. There was no pain, just a lot of pressure—maybe like a baby elephant sitting on top of my head.

It was the longest day of my life. I had been off my Parkinson medications since midnight the night before. I could not move. Even if I had been physically capable of moving, it was imperative that I remain motionless while the electrode was inside my brain mapping out the various structures.

Dr. DeLong has a unique way of explaining the mapping. It goes something like this: Imagine that your brain is like Europe, and the microelectrode is like a car. Just as one can drive across Europe in a car, so too can one drive across the brain with a microelectrode.

Many countries make up the continent of Europe, each country having certain landmarks, a specific language as well as purpose. As you drive across country borders from one country to another, you know what country you are in by its landmarks and its language. There are also many different regions in the brain, each region possessing unique landmarks—function and language. As the neurosurgeon drives the microelectrode down into the brain, the landmarks and the sounds (or language) that are heard in that region easily identify location.

The Pallidotomy team has a road map or atlas of the human brain to go by in order to help them determine location. However, each person's brain is unique and minor differences can make the difference between life and death in surgery. When performing a Pallidotomy, it is critical that the surgeon knows precisely which region of the brain the microelectrode is passing through. Mere millimeters separate the different regions, so, to be off by one or two millimeters can be devastating.

The Globus Pallidum is the region in the brain associated with movement disorder and Parkinson's disease, and it is located approximately 60 millimeters medially in the brain, resting just above the optic tract.

After five hours of mapping, I thought that I had reached my breaking point and absolutely could not stand it for one more minute. I clearly remember thinking to myself that it was horrible to have to endure such a grueling procedure by myself. I dared not interrupt Drs. DeLong and Vitek from their mapping because it was crucial to the outcome of the surgery. Besides, I had made a pact with the doctors before ever going into the operating room that no matter how hard it might become for me, I would endure it to the end. I lay on that table, amidst the chaos of the operating room, my head locked down to the table and an electrode sixty millimeters into my brain. It was then that I planned my future. While the doctors were mapping my brain, I was mapping out my future job as the Patient Support person for the Pallidotomy team. I would counsel with all prospective Pallidotomy patients, explaining to them exactly what to expect before, during, and following surgery. Additionally, I would be by their side in the operating room to be their emotional support, their eyes and ears, and to help them through the longest day of their lives.

At 3:00 PM, Dr. Bakay began the last stage of the Pallidotomy, the lesioning process. In the lesioning process, Dr. Bakay removed the microelectrode from the brain and in its place, inserted a probe whose tip was hot enough to fry an egg. By following the coordinates that Drs. Vitek and DeLong had mapped, he knew exactly which brain cells to kill. The very second that he touched the hot probe to the targeted brain cells, it felt as though someone had flipped a switch in my body. I underwent an immediate transformation from frozen, rigid, cramping, and immobile to feeling completely normal—like I felt in the years before Parkinson's disease. My outcome exceeded even the doctors' wildest dreams!

CNN took my story worldwide. Once my story was told, Emory's telephones started ringing, and they have not stopped since.

I did create the job I envisioned on the operating table. I participated in over 125 Pallidotomies and more than a dozen Deep Brain Stimulation cases in a four-year time span. I traveled nationwide, giving motivational speeches, and I lobbied in Congress for four years for the passage of the Morris K. Udall Bill for Parkinson's education and funding. I never again have asked God, "Why me?"

# ANGEL IN THE OR

There is a saying that, to paraphrase, says that some people come into our lives for a reason, some come for a season, and some come for a lifetime. I want to tell you about a person that I know in my heart came to me in a very special place, at a special time, for a special reason.

His name is Robert. Robert was an anesthesiologist at Emory University Hospital in 1993 when I had my Pallidotomy. Even though the operating room was filled to overflowing with people, and even though the day was all about me, all those many people each had a specific job to do in order for my procedure to be successful. There were the two neurologists, Dr. Vitek and Dr. DeLong, conducting the mapping of my brain; Dr. Mark Barron, assisting them; two more neurologists, Yoshi and Taca, visiting neurologists from Japan; and Dr. Rob Turner, PhD., monitoring the equipment; Dr. Bakay, the neurosurgeon, and his surgical resident, Dr. Cargill Allen. There were nurses assisting Dr. Bakay in prepping me for surgery, sterilizing instruments, and assisting him into his hospital scrubs. There was a doctor from Spain, Dr. Jose Obeso, there to observe the procedure that he intended to implement for his patients in Spain. Also seated at a table near the recording equipment were several people to chart every sound, movement, and any other activity that the recording and mapping of my brain would pick up. They charted every bit of activity on 3-dimensional maps.

Then, as if the room was not crowded enough, CNN had their camera crew with microphones, cameras, and special lights to film the Pallidotomy, as well as Rhonda Rowland, a reporter from CNN and the hospital PR representative, Lee Jenkins.

And then, off to my left side, amidst all the machines to monitor my vital signs, standing quietly by my side, rubbing my hand and offering me quiet, calm words of reassurance was Robert, my angel in the OR.

I learned much later that the role of the anesthesiologist in a Pallidotomy or a DBS (Deep Brain Stimulation) case is rather different from other surgical procedures. Generally, their role, in addition to monitoring vital signs, is to administer medications to keep the patient asleep during the procedure.

The anesthesiologist's role in a Pallidotomy case is quite the opposite. Unique for them, their job is simply to monitor vital signs, and to administer drugs, solely at the discretion of the neurologists and neurosurgeons. The point is that as a patient, I was to remain awake for the procedure. First, no Parkinson medication was given so as not to mask or control the symptoms. Secondly, they could not administer anesthesia because my active participation was crucial to the outcome of the Pallidotomy. Thirdly, pain medication had to be administered as sparingly as possible so that it would not alter the brain activity. Thus, Robert's role was necessary but limited. Yet, for me, he played one of the most important roles of all. He helped me get through the most agonizing day of my life.

There is no way I could have been adequately prepared for the feelings I would experience while locked down to the operating table, immobile, off medications, yet able to hear and see all that was taking place around me. It was a very long day. I was intensely uncomfortable, in mild to moderate pain, and terrified. I had complete faith in all the doctors—don't misunderstand me. However, when the lights went out and the mapping began, and all the noises that I couldn't see or understand began, it was overwhelming. Robert became my eyes, my ears, and my relaxation coach. When I became frightened or insecure, all I had to do was reach out my left hand, and he would find it and envelope it in his two warm hands, and rub my arm gently. At my request, he would stand up and look around trying to describe every sound made and every word spoken. This was his first Pallidotomy, too, so the experience was just as new for him as it was for me. I remember how kind and gentle he was. When I would feel close to reaching my breaking point and could go no further, he would sense that and cheer me on. "Just a few more minutes. They're almost finished. You can do it." One of the drugs allowable, sparingly, was for a headache, very mild and short acting. Imagine the headache you would have if you were in my place. All I had to do was mouth the word "headache" and within seconds, I would feel blissful relief. It lasted only minutes but was wonderful for the time.

Because my head was bolted down to the operating table, plus it was dark with the lights out and he was dressed in scrubs, a hat and mask, all I could see of him, when he leaned over me, was his incredibly beautiful blue eyes. They sparkled with gentleness and kindness. I knew that, although unable to see his hands, I would always remember the way they felt holding mine.

The next day I was still in ICU, waiting for transfer to a private room on the neurology wing of the hospital. A visitor appeared at the door to my cubicle. He didn't look familiar, yet I felt somehow I knew him. He said he was in the OR with me the day before and just wanted to see how I was doing. The voice was sounding familiar now. As he came closer, I could see his eyes. "Come here and let me hold your hand," I said to him. I shut my eyes as he approached the bed and took my hand in his. I smiled, opening my eyes again. "Robert! Thank you for yesterday, for being my support." He just smiled, squeezed my hand gently, and quietly left the room.

I worked at Emory for over four years, 1993–1997. I participated in close to 150 procedures, encountering many anesthesiologists, some of them, frequently. I never saw Robert again.

# MOUTH OF THE SOUTH

As I have stated earlier, there are times in our lives when we meet some people for a reason, others for a season, and still others for a lifetime. The first time I ever saw Joan Samuelson was in 1992 on CNN. She was testifying before Congress regarding the grossly inadequate funding for Parkinson's disease research. I remember exactly where I was, what I was doing, and how I felt. I was sitting in my recliner in my house in Sandersville watching TV, or rather, I was flipping through the channels. I had recently retired on total disability and was thinking about what I would do with the rest of my life. I was depressed, and it was difficult to think about a future when I was still trying to reconcile the fact that I could no longer work because of the symptoms of Parkinson's disease that haunted me constantly.

Something about the way she was standing before the podium caught my eye, so I paused and watched her testimony for a few minutes. Imagine my surprise when I found out that she, too, had Parkinson's disease. At that time, I did not know a single living soul in my age group with Parkinson's disease. Suddenly appearing on my TV was a young, attractive, vibrant woman speaking passionately about the need for more money from Congress to fund research for Parkinson's disease. Why did it suddenly make me feel better to see her? For the first time since my diagnosis, I didn't feel all alone with my disease. She exhibited some of the same symptoms I did, and there she was—an attorney who had lost her practice and her marriage to the disease—speaking passionately and intelligently about her experiences. She didn't look or sound crazy, and she didn't appear to feel sorry for herself.

"Well, my goodness," I thought, "There are other people in the world fighting the same battle as I. There really is life after Parkinson's disease." I wished that the day would come when I could meet her, talk to her, and find out more about her personal mission. Little did I know...Not quite two years later, after my successful Pallidotomy, I was working at Emory University with the Pallidotomy team of doctors as the patient support advocate.

I received some information in the mail one day advertising PAN's (Parkinson Action Network) annual forum in Washington, D.C. Reading the literature, it sounded like something that would be informative, interesting, and a way to use my social and speaking skills to help promote public awareness about Parkinson's disease.

I showed the information to Dr. DeLong, and he agreed that I should attend the annual forum in Washington, D.C. That was the beginning of six years of political advocacy. Four years were spent making many trips to Washington and finally moving there for a year. I joined a grassroots group of People with Parkinson's disease under the auspices of PAN, whose leader was none other than Joan Samuelson. Talk about a wish coming true! I learned how to visit with U.S. Representatives and Senators and tell my own story, as well as to ask for their support in the passage of a bill, named for the late congressional member, Morris K. Udall, who died from complications related to Parkinson's disease. The bill was asking for a fair distribution of funding for medical research by increasing that for Parkinson's disease. Washington is where I met, worked with, and came to love, so dearly, many people from all over the country who had one thing in common. We either all had Parkinson's disease or we loved someone dearly who had Parkinson's disease.

We laughed together. We cried together. We shared our meals, our medication, and our sorrows, always ending the night by splurging on hot fudge sundaes on the rooftop of the Hotel Washington, our home away from home. This is where we would meet after a long, grueling, emotional day on the Hill to laugh, cry, and boast of our triumphs of the day.

There was Jim Cordy, nicknamed, "The General"; Carol Walton in her perfect "Princess Di" suits; and Mary Yost, our behind the scenes scheduler from sunny California, without whom we would never have found the right Senator in the right office at the right time in the right building. How did she work her magic? By waking up at 3 AM, she could start calling the switchboard on Capital Hill at 4 AM, PST. She was our cheerleader and the surprise giver of great fruit baskets, flowers, champagne, and a constant flow of encouragement.

We each had our own distinct flair when it came to trying to woo the votes and promises of votes from the Congressmen. Carol's approach was to confidently march into the office of a senator wearing her flawless "Princess Di" suit of the day, with her perfect hair, her flawless makeup, and beautifully manicured nails. With rapid fire, she would spout out data of the proposed Bill, not unlike a car salesperson trying to sell a Lexus. She was a salesperson to the core.

Margy's approach was different. While Carol was speaking on behalf of her father, who had suffered for years in a nursing home before dying from complications of Parkinson's, Margy did an absolutely brilliant job of showing the House Majority Leader exactly what Parkinson's disease looked like. She is very tall, almost 6 feet, and slender with excellent verbal skills. She walks with the aid of a mountain climbing staff. If there were advantages to having Parkinson's disease, it would be the ability to show Congress the violent, cruel ways that Parkinson's disease ravages the body. The ace in her pocket was to quit taking her medication about an hour before the scheduled visit. Her tall, statuesque body would literally be aquiver with tremors, imbalanced and stumbling. That image burns in the brains of anyone who sees her.

Lupe, with her no nonsense approach, probably stemming from her psychiatric nursing background as well as her fiery Latino personality, had yet a different style. She would simply stand firmly planted in the Representative's office, with her hands on her hips, and state sternly, "I will not take no for an answer. It is simply not acceptable."

Then there was my approach. I was the physically demonstrative, emotional one. I was also the cheerleader of the group. The first thing I would do, unconventionally, upon walking in the offices of our distinguished Congressmen was to bypass their outstretched hand and zoom in for a big hug. That usually caught them off guard. I would always have done my homework and found the name, address, and telephone number of at least one constituent within their district that had Parkinson's disease, and I would tell the Congressman that I was there on his constituent's behalf. "He would have been here instead of me if it was possible, but the medications that he must take to control his symptoms are so expensive that he couldn't afford the trip. Nor could he navigate through the halls of Congress. He also cannot speak well enough for others to understand him. Therefore, I am here to speak for those who can no longer speak for themselves. I am also here to show you proof of the dramatic difference the research dollar made in my life."

It was NIH funding, such that was available at the time, that made the Pallidotomy program possible and ultimately successful. When the Congressman stood to shake our hands and thanked us for stopping by, he did not extend his hand towards me. He just braced himself, ready for the hug that he knew was coming.

There was also Bob and Nancy, Mort and Millie, Perry, Vernice, Pat, Susan and Stan, and the General's wife, Deborah. Who could forget Ken, Saul, or Mike? Some of the people would come and go over the years. Others were there for the long haul.

I will never forget the way I obtained the support and vote from Senator Sam Nunn, Senator from my home state of Georgia. I tried unsuccessfully to see him on several occasions in his office. On my weekly early Monday morning flight to Washington from Atlanta, we had been in the air for only a few minutes when I turned from my aisle seat and saw Senator Nunn walking up the aisle. At that point, I did not stop and think through what my actions should be. I was just so excited to see him, finally, that all I could think about was getting to him so I could get his support for our bill. Without thinking, I jumped up from my seat and stepped in the aisle in front of him. Nervously, and what seemed to be all in one breath, I said, "Senator Nunn, I'm sorry to bother you, but I have been trying to get an appointment with you for weeks and keep missing you. My name is Terrie Whitling. I am from Georgia, and I have Parkinson's disease. I am visiting all of the Georgia congressional representatives asking for their vote on the Morris K. Udall Bill to increase funding for Parkinson's Research. Will you support the bill and vote yes when it comes to vote?"

If I startled Senator Nunn, he was very gracious and regained his composure very quickly. He assured me that he knew of the bill and intended to support it. I was so excited that I threw myself at him, almost knocking him down with my powerful hug. He just laughed as he straightened himself back up. I was so embarrassed when I sat back down in my seat. I had just attacked a Senator on the airplane! Moreover, to make matters worse, I had gotten lipstick on the collar of his freshly starched, light blue oxford shirt. I sure hope he did not notice.

A memorable visit of a different nature comes to mind. Walking the halls of the House and Senate buildings was hard for healthy people and could be anywhere from grueling to impossible for people with Parkinson's. One day, I had agreed to go with friends, Lyn Coles and Mike Clippinger, to visit their district's representative from Indiana. It had been a tiring morning for me. By the time we had walked to the representative's office, my Parkinson's disease demanded attention, as I completely froze in the hallway just before the door to his office. The secretary found a chair for me to sit in because I could not walk, and I was rapidly becoming unable to speak. I convinced Lyn and Mike to go to the meeting without me. I would stay in the hall until my medication kicked in and then I would join them. When my medications wear off, I can become paranoid at other people watching me, so I asked Lyn to face me towards the wall so no one would look at me. The meeting with the representative ended up in the hall. Without trying, I may have made the biggest impression, as the representative could clearly see first-hand how disabling the disease is and how quickly one can go from walking and talking to total immobility.

PAN has had many successes over the years. The one that I was a part of was the successful passage of the Morris K. Udall Bill for Education and Research. It passed in October 1997, after four long years.

It was here that I earned my nicknames and wore them with honor. I am known in certain exclusive circles as the, "Mouth of the South." "The General" bestowed this title of honor and the following one upon me—I was their, "Queen of Dixie." The people may have drifted apart, but the nicknames remained. So did the love and respect we had for each other.

# SMALL TOWN

As an adult, one of the nicest aspects of growing up in a small town is in knowing practically everyone in town. As a child, one of the worst aspects of growing up in a small town is that practically everyone in the town knew me. That also meant that practically everyone knew my parents. This known fact meant that I could not get away with anything. Somebody that knew my family would always be watching me. My parents warned me that no matter what I did, no matter where I was, they would find out about it. Those were not just idle threats either. It took me far too long to realize that they were right. Wherever I was, whatever I was doing, if it was wrong, you can bet that before nightfall, our telephone would start ringing with a well-meaning friend of my parents calling to tell on me.

Is this what Hilary meant in her book, *It Takes a Village to Raise a Child*? My villagers sure had their eyes on me. Those same eyes were on me as I grew up, moved away, married, and moved back home to start my family. They were still on me when I divorced, as well as when I enrolled in college and when I developed Parkinson's disease.

One has to take the good with the bad in a small town that knows you. No one in my small hometown had ever seen a young person with Parkinson's disease. But, neither had I. If they had, they didn't recognize it because its "face" can be very deceiving. There wasn't anyone to compare me to. There was only, "Old Man Todd." All who knew him referred to his shaking palsy as "Saint Vitas Dance." His movements were erratic and jerky, causing his head to move in peculiar ways and his arms and legs to "dance" out of control. We all knew to get the hell out of his way, and fast, if we saw him driving down the road in his old,

49

black Edsel. He drove just as he walked, with the same kind of "dancing" down the road. He would weave from one side of the road to the other. Often, he would end up either on the sidewalk or in someone's bushes. No one knew, at the time, that he and I were actually suffering from the same disease. Until my small town and I became better educated, there would be whispers behind my back—"She is on drugs, I hear." "Does she have a drinking problem?" and sometimes, not so quietly, "She must be nuts!"

It took a while for us all to become educated in the different "faces" of Parkinson's disease. We fear that which we do not understand. The comfort level, for me, in my hometown, is that everybody knew me "before."

Small town living has its blessings, too. In 1993, I underwent the first of several brain surgeries to alleviate worsening symptoms of Parkinson's disease. I was on every prayer list in every church in the county. I received hundreds of get-well cards from Sunday school classes I never attended and from people I knew only by their family name.

The local people couldn't spell or pronounce Pallidotomy, nor could they explain the benefits it would provide for me. They cared for me enough to pray for me, though, because I was one of theirs. They cared enough to educate themselves through local newspaper articles written about me and by me. Once they had seen its "face" and could give it a name, Parkinson's disease, I could return to who I had always been behind the "face"—ME.

I live in a different small town now and have a different last name. In many ways, it is much like my hometown. I feel the stares and hear the whispers behind my back. At times, I feel like an alien. I understand the stares and whispers though. The people in this small town did not know me "before"… They know only what they see now. I guess they do not know the many faces of Parkinson's disease. Maybe I should introduce myself.

# THE MANY FACES OF PARKINSON'S DISEASE

During the year that I lived in Washington, D.C., I continued to commute to Atlanta to help with the Pallidotomy cases. One memorable case was with a 52-year-old man, a former body builder and real estate tycoon from New Jersey. His was a very interesting case and subsequently, we became good friends. More importantly, I was fascinated and fell in love with his mother and his daughters. She was a very strong, independent woman, in her late seventies but looking a good twenty years younger than her age. A strong friendship developed between us, too. There was becoming less and less need for my staying in Washington. I began visiting my new friends at their home in New Jersey and eventually was invited to move in with them. They quickly welcomed me into their family, and the mother made me feel like the daughter she'd never had. I moved into the house with her son, and slowly, over time, became his companion and caregiver. This was a life that would consume me for the next three years— 1997–1999.

Like everything else in my life, I believe I was there for a reason. Following this introduction is a very lengthy account of life with Parkinson's disease and the many faces that it showed as time went on:

*This is a true and accurate retelling of a conversation I had several years ago with a friend, who like myself, has battled with Parkinson's disease. I dedicate this chapter in memory of my friend, George Rollin Parker III, who recently passed away after battling this monster of a disease for more than 20 years.*

"Do you know what time it is? Get up!" said Rol excitedly, waking me from a very deep sleep. I sat up in the recliner, groggily, where I had fallen asleep at 11:30 PM, just a few hours earlier. "Look at the clock! Do you see what time it is?" he determinedly continued. The clock was to my back. I awakened extremely stiff and unable to turn my head.

"I can't see it, Rol. Look for me and tell me what time it is."

"It's 8:30," he said with confidence. You need to get up."
arms out to Rol. With his help, slowly, painfully I unfolded myself from the deep crevices of the recliner, stretching and moaning with pain as I stood. A little wobbly, I gingerly turned my head to look at the clock behind me. "It's only 2:30 AM, I groaned. Go back to bed".

By this time, Rol was in the kitchen cutting brownies left over from dinner earlier in the evening. Piling them high on a plate, he began licking his fingers, sticky with chocolate from the icing. Smearing some of the icing on the front of his tee shirt, he began talking rapidly in a familiar yet undecipherable gibberish. It was enough to alert me to the fact that, despite outward appearances, he was not awake. He was in, what I had come to know, one of the many faces of Parkinson's disease. It is common, in the more animated faces, for him to go on food forages during the night. The key factor is to understand that he is not necessarily awake. He has one foot in reality and one foot in dreamland. I, too, have one foot in reality and one foot in dreamland, as I become a part of his dream through our verbal exchange.

I have found, from experience, that two specific questions, reliably, help me to determine his reality state.

"Are you awake?" I ask.

"No, I'm not awake. Not for wrestling, anyway" he replied very coherently. This question, as well as the answer, may sound silly to some. I find it very helpful, though, as Rol, most likely, will be up, walking and talking, with his eyes wide open. If one didn't know better, one would think he was awake, lucid and carrying on a perfectly normal conversation. One clue to the contrary is that this conversation was taking place at two o'clock in the morning. The second clue is that Rol is completely honest, awake or asleep. I am sure he has told a lie or two in his life but he doesn't hide it very well.

Before I could ask the second question; "Do you know who I am?" Rol attempted to ask me for something. He couldn't find the words to verbalize what he wanted. We played 20 questions until I finally deciphered that he wanted some lemonade similar to what we had for dinner, earlier that night.

"We're out of canned lemonade, but I can mix some powered lemonade for you."

"I would like that. Thank you," Rol replied sweetly.

The next part of our conversation took place in the kitchen at 2 AM while Rol dropped crumbs all over the floor trying to eat his fistful of brownies. I was simply trying to stay awake, find the lemonade mix, and decipher the conversation that follows:

Rol: "Tell me something. Were you the valedictorian of your class or was Bill Clinton?"

Me: "It wasn't me."

Rol: Was it Bill Clinton, then?"

Me: "I don't know. I didn't go to Georgetown."

Rol: "Yes, you did."

Me: "No, Rol, I didn't go to Georgetown."

Rol: "Then you can't be Bill Clinton."

Me: "That's right. I'm not Bill Clinton. Do you know who I am?"

Rol: "Well, if you didn't go to Georgetown and you're not Bill Clinton, maybe you're George Rollin Parker the 'TURD.'"

Unless you know what transpired earlier that day, you surely are shaking you head in bewilderment by now. Rol had received a telephone call earlier in the day from Lew, a childhood friend of his. Lew, now a prominent physician in Arlington, Virginia, was in Bill Clinton's graduating class at Georgetown. Rumor has it that Bill Clinton claims to have been valedictorian of his graduating class. Oddly enough, Lew said he remembered the valedictorian. His name wasn't Bill Clinton.

For the second time I asked, "Are you awake?"

Rol: "No, but I'm a nice boy. I won't hurt you."

Me: "Do you know who I am?"

A puzzled look on his face, shaking his head, he replied in a voice, so soft, barely more than a whisper. "I don't think so." His speech, clear for the past few minutes, again became garbled. Picking up his plate of brownies in one hand, his urinal in the other, (when Rol had first come out to the living room to awaken me, he had brought with him his urinal with fresh urine and set it on the kitchen counter next to the brownies). He shuffled toward his bedroom.

Rol: "Goodnight, Mom."

Me: "I'm not your mother."

Rol: "Okay, I don't know who you are."

After depositing the contents of the urinal in the bathroom, Rol went back to the kitchen for his lemonade. When he reached his bed, he dropped the lemonade, spilling it all over the floor. Hitting the wall with his fists, he screamed, "Damn, #&@^*$ this mess! G-damn shit!"

In reality, Rol is a very mild-mannered man. He does not use his fists in any way and rarely speaks profanely. Damn, on occasion, sure, but never the other words. It just isn't in his nature. The outburst focuses solely on him but is quite violent. This was the first time I had seen this display of violence in an otherwise gentle man.

"It's okay. It's no big deal. It's only lemonade. You go back to sleep. It will only take a minute to clean this up."

I guided him back to his bed, which was simply a mattress on the floor. I helped him down to the floor, first changing his shirt, washing his hands, adjusting his sheet and pillow, rinsed out his urinal, placing it within arm's reach, and finally, cleaned up the spilled lemonade.

Later, when Rol was more lucid and verbal, we discussed the episode I just described.

Rol said, "I remember all of this," referring to my recount of the 2:30 episode. "Understand, though, it wasn't you I was talking to when I asked if you were the Valedictorian. When I looked at you, it was Lew I saw, not you. I was talking to Lew. When I said 'Goodnight Mom,' it was my mother I saw standing in the hall, not you. It is scary when I read this recount. On one hand, I want to laugh. I think, who is this comedian writing this stuff? This is good stuff. Then I realize that it's no comedian. It is me, it's real, and it's not always funny. Most of the time it's very scary."

"I remember the time I attacked you while I was having a night terror."

"I remember that night vividly," I said. It was the first time I had ever seen or heard you in that face, or catatonic state. I heard you moaning 'help me, help me' repeatedly. I ran downstairs to see what was wrong and found you lying flat on the floor on your stomach. When I tried to move you, I found that you were completely rigid, almost paralyzed and catatonic, yet you continued to chant 'help me, help me' in a monotone kind of moan. It was like trying to lift dead weight. As I exerted more effort in trying to help you up, it was as though a switch flipped in your brain. Suddenly, with a rush of adrenaline, you jumped up off the floor, grabbed me around my knees, and flipped me up in the air, over the recliner in your bedroom, and I landed on the floor. Not only did it hurt, but also it scared the hell out of me. I had never encountered anything like that in my life!"

Rol replied, "It frightens me to think that it could happen again. To live this way every day and never know when it is going to happen or what it will be like. I am afraid when people read this; they will think I am a monster! Do you understand now that I was dreaming that I was in a war, and I thought you were the enemy trying to kill me? I was defending myself.

"Did I really use the F word? That is so embarrassing for anyone to read. What will they think of me? I don't mind the 'damn' so much…"

The above dialogue is one brief example of another face of Parkinson's disease—the Rol of days gone by, the "normal" Rol, the Rol that everyone in his small town remembers and speaks of lovingly. He is articulate, clear-minded, alert, intelligent, witty, sensitive, and caring. To look at him at this moment, you would never suspect that he has Parkinson's disease. His voice is clear, strong, and intelligible, ; his face is fully animated. There is no sign of dyskinesia, tremor, gait disturbance, freezing, mental confusion, or any other symptom of the disease. He is strong, independent, and confident—looking at least ten years younger. Those clear, twinkling, blue eyes, quick and alert; that irresistible smile; clapping his hands and rubbing them together as he becomes more and more excited in our conversation. This face, quite naturally, is my favorite. However brief or infrequently this face shows itself, it far outshines all the others. It is this face that motivates me to work and educate and advocate for this disease. Hopefully, one day, in the near future, neither Rol nor I will have to bear this hideous disease. This face keeps me here, wanting to see it more.

On other days, another face shines through.

I walked in Rol's bedroom to find him down on his hands and knees, writing on the carpet with his finger. He appeared to be concentrating very hard on whatever it was that he was writing.

"What are you doing on the floor?" I asked.

"I'm figuring the luxury tax," he said, without looking up.

"What luxury tax?" I asked, curious.

"On that hotel over there," he said, pointing across the room. "Have you seen the file on it?"

"No, "I haven't seen it. Rol, are you awake?"

"No I'm not," he stated, clearly and matter of fact.

"I wish you were awake."

"I wish I were awake, too, but I have to finish this tax. I need the file from the desk." With that said, he got up from the floor, walked to the kitchen, opened the pantry door, and took out the box of Raisin Bran cereal. Holding it high for me to see, he asked, "Is this the file?" Not waiting for an answer, he proceeded to fix himself a bowl of cereal and began, ravenously, to devour it.

"Are you awake yet?" I asked, as I sat down at the table just opposite him.

"I think so," he replied haltingly.

"Who am I, then?"

With a puzzled look on his face, he said, "I'm not sure."

We sat quietly at the table together as I watched him eat his cereal. For the third time I asked, "Do you know who I am?"

Finally, "I think I do."

"What is my name?"

His face underwent a complete transformation, instantly becoming much clearer and more alert. "Oh, you're Terrie."

It is interesting to me that once Rol is awake, lucid and able to articulate, he usually remembers the conversations from his dream state. He can usually clarify the dream for me, and I can usually find a common thread from an earlier discussion of that topic while he is in reality.

Immediately after the latest early morning conversation with Rol, I rushed to my computer while it was still fresh in my mind. I wanted to capture the episode on paper. By this time, though, it was 4:30 AM. My thoughts were clear; the words were ready to go from my fingers to the computer. My body, however, was rebelling against the work before me. I was slowing down, physically, with severe cramping, painful, in my left shoulder. My gait was slow with short, shuffling steps. I took a Sinemet, but I knew it wouldn't take effect for a while, yet. I felt that I couldn't afford to wait until the Sinemet began to work. I wanted to write this while it was still so fresh in my mind. My typing was very slow and spastic. I had tremendous difficulty in hitting the correct keys. I quickly decided that if I worried about typographical errors, misspelled words, dangling participles or split infinitives, I would NEVER finish it. I would do the best I could, given the circumstances, and clean it up later.

I finally finished around 5:30 AM. I stumbled back to bed for one more hour of much needed sleep. Rol came upstairs and woke me at 6:30, reminding me that I had a 9:00 appointment with the chiropractor. When I first awakened, I was completely stiff; my movements were in slow motion, and it felt like every part of my body hurt. It hurt to move my back. It hurt not to move it, too. I peeled myself off the bed, shuffled, slowly, painfully into the kitchen in search of my first dose of Sinemet, Mirapex, coffee, and Zoloft—in that hierarchy of needs. My speech is intelligible at this early hour, but very soft in volume. My words tend to slur more until the first dose of Sinemet kicks in.

I know by the poor response I'm having to the Sinemet that it's going to be a challenging morning. Rol is having a similarly poor response to his medication. It is apparent by his turtle-like movements that shaving, for him, this morning, is not going to be an option. If I were having a better morning, I would shave him myself, as I seem to be doing more and more lately; however, I am too shaky to be trusted with a razor in my hand today.

Rol is going with me to the chiropractor's appointment. It will take every spare minute between 6:30 and 9:00 AM to get myself showered, fed, and dressed, then to see that Rol gets in and out of the shower safely. He fell twice while I was upstairs taking a shower. Lately, he falls daily. So far, the worst of his injuries are a bruised left knee and a bruised ego.

Once I finished dressing, I helped Rol dress—he was too far "off" to do it himself. I pulled his underpants up over a still damp butt, only partially dried after his shower. Next to go on was his knit shirt. My balance was poor now. I had to fight to keep from falling as I reached up to pull the shirt over his head. When I reached my arms over his head, my shoulders began to cramp. I had to stop and work out cramps before I could finish dressing him. I realized that my breathing was very shallow, panting almost. I concentrated on breathing deep, cleansing breaths to help work through the pain. Looking at the clock, I saw it was already 8:40.

There was very little talking going on between us, as it was taking full concentration, for both of us, just to get dressed and out the door. There was still so much to do, so much to remember. I had to finish dressing Rol, help him walk to the car, be sure I had a "to go" drink for the car, our medication, Rol's glasses, my pocketbook, jackets for both of us, car keys, house keys. Did I remember to lock the house?

Once Rol was in the car, I remembered that I'd left the grocery list and coupons on the kitchen counter. The pain had not subsided, so I walked slowly and painfully back to the house for the forgotten items. Damn, I thought. Will my medication ever kick in?

Back in the car with Rol, both of us strapped in our seat belts, I drove slowly out of the driveway as Rol tried to help me stretch out my shoulder muscles to relieve the pain. Finally, the medications began to work. As they did so, my feet began turning inward in a rigid, cramping (dystonic) action. From experience, I knew the foot dystonia was only fleeting. It did make for difficult driving, though.

At 9:03, we were just pulling out onto the divided highway. Obviously, we were gong to be late. I hate being late. The unpredictability of the disease drives me nuts, I think to myself, as I pass another half of a Sinemet to Rol. He still had not "turned on."

At the chiropractor's office, finally, I got my first lucky break—an empty parking space right next to the door. Hurrying around to Rol's side of the car, I pulled him up and out of the car, all 200 pounds of him, pressed his baseball cap down on his head, hiding the cowlick on the top of his head. I did not have time to comb his hair, and he still couldn't do it either.

"Watch my foot, Rol. Take your time. We're not in any hurry. That's right. Take a big step. Think about what you're doing. You're doing great! Slow down! You're going too fast, pitching yourself forward. Stand up straight, take a deep breath. Great, now look at my foot and take a step."

I left Rol in the waiting room while I went in for my appointment. The people there love him very much, so I know I don't have to worry about him. Back in the car about 30 minutes later, Rol still hadn't turned on. I gave him another half of Sinemet. I ran a short errand before going to the grocery store hoping to give him time to turn on so that he could help me buy groceries. It didn't work. At the grocery store, he stayed in the car while I went in. Five minutes later, I looked up to find Rol running down the aisle towards me, throwing the car keys ahead of him on the floor so that they slid towards me. There was that wicked grin of his, again, and a twinkle in his eye. He's back! Such is the nature of this hideous disease.

It is the drugs, the years of abusing Sinemet, that is partially to blame for the many faces. Just a few years ago, Rol was under the care of a very prominent, world-renowned movement disorder specialist who said to him, "Take as much Sinemet as you need to be functional." Well, Rol, no different from any other person with Parkinson's disease, didn't like the way it felt to be out of control, unable to move when he wanted to. The Sinemet, for a while, gave him that control back, but at the expense of taking increasingly larger and larger doses as time went on. No one ever told him about the long-term side effects. The period I am referring to is recent when we all knew about dyskinesia, when we all knew about short-term memory loss, when we all knew about hallucinations. The doctor that gave him carte Blanc on Sinemet intake has written a book, for God's sake, about Parkinson's disease. Until recently, he was taking 300mgs of Sinemet every 1½ hours. It was not uncommon for him to take up to 20 Sinemet tablets during the night. No wonder he has permanent memory loss. No wonder he has night terrors. No wonder he has so many faces.

I probably should distinguish between the many faces, as they each have very distinct visual, psychological, physical, and personality characteristics. I realize this is beginning to sound like *The Three Faces of Eve*. I don't want to imply that I think Rol suffers from Dissociative Disorder. You will see what I mean about the uniqueness of each face. It is because Parkinson's disease has multiple faces that the disease is so complex, so misunderstood. Let me see if I can write a picture of the different faces of Rol.. Let me add, too, that I don't believe that Rol is unique in his many faces. I believe that all of us who suffer from this disease have our own individual combination of many faces.

First face – I see the man, the child, the boy before Parkinson's disease. He is whole; he is independent, in control, confident, successful, and articulate. He is a leader. He is a million-dollar salesperson, a successful real estate broker. He is an athlete. He is strong and powerful. He runs races and wins. He flies like the wind in his speedboat. He is sure of foot and swift of mind. He pumps iron with energy and vitality. He is sensitive and sentimental. He cries at Lone Ranger shows and watches the Disney channel with child-like glee. He is a tease, a flirt, and yet, the perfect gentleman. He is steady as a rock with the memory of an elephant, the stamina of a horse, and a heart of gold.

Second face –I see the man, the child, the boy disabled. He is fearful, insecure, and dependent. His knee is permanently discolored from the bruising that occurs from his daily falls. He shuffles and shakes. He is weak, unable to open his can of coke. He is flat, depressed, and hopeless. He can't remember what day it is, what he had for breakfast, if he even had breakfast. He is afraid of the dark and of things that go bump in the night. He cries for help to go to the bathroom to dress him, and, at times, to feed him. He looks both very old and yet acts very childlike. He hates this face and would like to keep it hidden from the world. Wouldn't you?

The third face is one of the hardest ones to describe to someone that has never seen it. Let me describe the following scenario:

Rol and I have been working on his "Christmas Letter" since December 1st. It's turned into somewhat of a joke that we still haven't finished it. Maybe, with any luck, we'll have it finished by next Christmas. Several days ago, he expressed an interest in working on it. Several years ago, he wouldn't have needed my help, or anyone's, for that matter, to write his letters for him. He was a gifted writer, in his own right, with a strong command of the English language. Words came to him easily. He spoke with ease. He wrote with equal ease. He knew spelling, he knew definition, and he knew grammar.

I believe that Parkinson's disease attacks us at the core of our beings. It robs us of our unique talents, skill, and passion. This is certainly true for Rol. Although Rol needs help with the mechanics of writing, I want the words and thoughts to be his own, not mine. His concentration is such that we can work on it only for a few minutes at a time. Thinking, perhaps, this morning would be a good time to work on it, hopefully to finish it, I copied what we had done so far and took it downstairs looking for Rol. I found him on the living room floor writhing uncontrollably. I was wondering how to show the third face. Of all the faces, the third face is the most frustrating to me. Unlike the others, I am unsure of how, when, or why it occurs. When he shows this face, the 3rd face, he is clearly misunderstood by those who encounter him. Unless they know him, they mistake him for a drunk, a drug addict, or someone with psychiatric problems. It is what I call his "goofy" look. He hates people to see him in this state.

Most people with Parkinson's take Sinemet striving for relief from the rigid, frozen state of Parkinson's. At some point, Rol, sometimes from taking too much medication, sometimes from a buildup of medication over time and sometimes for no viable reason, overreacts from the rigid, frozen state. He has movement, which is certainly preferable to the frozen, akinetic state. In this face, however, he has too much movement, equally uncontrollable. In an effort to regain control over the movement of his body, he is still out of control!

In the second face, Rol's' speech is low, slow, and unintelligible. In the third face, his speech is too fast, with his words running together, equally unintelligible.

"This is very frustrating for me," says Rol, as he lies on the living room floor, left arm and leg flailing about uncontrollably as though they are separate entities, with lives of their own.

"Why are you talking with your eyes closed?" I asked. Rol shakes his head repeatedly, back and forth, in frustration, his eyebrows furrowed, eyes clenched tightly shut.

"I'm trying to concentrate—so I can make the words come out right," he said haltingly. "This is so hard! When I'm like this, I can't remember anything either. When I try to write my name, I can't remember even how to spell it." He hits his head with the heel of his hand in frustration. He is to the point of tears. "It just won't work like I want it to."

"When you are like this, do you have the thoughts you want to express in your brain and yet, you can't get them in the right order and out of your mouth in a coherent fashion?"

"Yes! That's exactly it!" cried Rol.

"Tell me more about how you feel."

"I feel so weak right now that I don't think I can even get up off the floor. There is no energy (within me)."

"Would you like me to tell you exactly how you look right now?"

"I'm not sure if I want to hear this…." He paused. "Okay. Tell me."

"You look just like a drunk, homeless person straight out of one of the parks in D.C. You have this goofy look on your face, and your head is cocked over to one side. I've noticed that when you try to walk, you look limp as a marionette, rather disjointed and always leaning far over to one side. You have a great deal of trouble sitting straight in a chair. All the movement throws you to the floor. I have seen you eat many a meal half in the chair and half on the floor."

"Yes, I know how it looks, but I can't help it! I hate it! I know, now, why you can't understand me when my speech is messed up as it is now. Remember the other day when I heard myself on the tape recorder? I could not even understand myself! It was terrible. I had no idea I sounded that bad! I am still concerned about what people will think of me if they hear me say those terrible words I said the other night. I don't want to make up anything that doesn't really happen, but I don't want people to think I am really the kind of person that normally talks like that."

"Did I ever tell you about my friend, the retired Baptist preacher from South Carolina, who had brain surgery a few years ago when I was working at Emory University?"

"I can't remember if you have or not."

"Well, he was proof that everyone has a breaking point. A soft-spoken, mild-mannered man under normal circumstances, he reached the bewitching hour in surgery when his anxiety was so great that he became very combative, striking out at both the doctor and me. He said all the same words you said. He said them in front of about 15 people in the operating room. I coined the phrase 'SDH Syndrome'—that point in time during the surgery when the patient thinks he cannot go any further. For my preacher friend, his breaking point was to shout 'shit, damn, hell.' Anyone who knows him, though, knows that he's not a SDH kind of guy any more than you are."

"I think it's the disease talking. It's the frustration of the disease," Rol said.

"When I read back over everything I've written about the many faces of Parkinson's disease, it strikes me very hard that several of the faces have shown themselves within the past 24 hours—not just once but many times. What I think is important for you to remember, Rol, is that you represent the community of People with Parkinson's disease. We all have the many faces of Parkinson's disease. We exhibit them differently, and to greater and lesser degrees, but we all must struggle with the constant ebb and flow as each face presents itself and then backs away, lending room for the next face to appear. I have the many faces, too.

No wonder we have no energy. No wonder we can't sleep. No wonder we're depressed. For those people who are afraid of merry-go-rounds, ferris wheels, and roller coasters, it is no wonder they leave their loved ones who have Parkinson's disease. Parkinson's disease never sleeps. It never takes a vacation. It never even takes a day off. It is never ceasing. At times, it is a living hell.

# *IN THE BOAT*

If I could make time stand still, it would be the times when my friend, Rol, is in his boat on Lake Wallenpaupack, in the Poconoes. It is amazing to watch his transformation! The Parkinson's disease that has ravaged his body, his mind and at times, his spirit, miraculously disappears! He looks like a normal, healthy, physically unimpaired man. His voice is strong, his movements steady and sure, his face relaxed. His confidence is solid as a rock and all his fear is gone. Rol is in control!

Those of us who live with Parkinson's disease know that emotions, stress, and our psychological state of well-being all play a significant role in the symptoms manifested as well as the severity of the symptoms. The more positively we react to the situations, the less impact potential stressors will have on the disease. Just come watch Rol in his boat, if you don't believe me.

Rol's boat is no ordinary boat, mind you. It is a speedboat—a sleek, blue beauty capable of going 80 mph. Very few boats on Lake Wallenpaupack compare with this boat. For that matter, very few people on Lake Wallenpaupack compare with the driver of this boat.

Now, I love to drive my car. I am confident when I drive, and I am not afraid to drive fast because I know that I am a good driver. It was not until I drove Rol's boat that I could appreciate the strength, the confidence, and steadiness it takes to drive a boat like that. I was not confident driving it. I did not feel in control. The boat was the power, and it controlled me. Then Rol took over and the change in him was immediate. He was the power, in control, confident and steady. While he was behind the wheel of his boat, his Parkinson's disease was gone.

I had a conversation with Mike, a friend of Rol's. A college roommate, Mike, 52, was looking forward to retiring from the army soon. "I can't wait to take Rol to the Poconoes so we can take his boat out. It's been years since we've been able to do that. Maybe we can even ski. Have you seen Rol ski?" asked Mike.

"No, but I've heard the stories of his 'fabulous feat of the feet'; the best skier on Cranberry Lake, they say. Is it true that he could ski barefoot?"

"It's true all right. I've seen him do it. Rol is amazing! The last time I saw him on skis was three years ago."

"You're kidding," I exclaimed. "I thought it was 10 or 15 years ago since he skied."

"No, it was just three years. I was up in the Poconoes with him. I pulled him in his boat. He couldn't start off on one ski, but he dropped it after he was up and soon after, he dropped the other one. It was something to see. I saw him go from being unable to get out of the car without help, unable to walk to his boat without help. He even needed help to put his skis on. Once he jumped into the water though, he was like a different person. He could ski barefoot!"

What mysteries the brain holds!

# CARDS IN THE WIND

I grew up in a family of card players—at least 3 generations, maybe more. Just name the game and I can play it—Gin, Rummy, Poker, Spades, Hearts, Canasta, etc. Playing cards is just one of those things that come naturally, I guess.

My sister, Gail, and I have been life-long Spade partners, as well as Gin opponents. How I wish I had kept a record of the number of games, the years, the score that we played over the past 25–30 years.

During my travels public speaking, fund raising, and working in political advocacy for Parkinson's disease, I noticed an elderly couple sitting in one of the waiting areas in the Miami airport. I could tell from where I was standing, 20 feet away, that they were playing cards. I had a little time, as I was waiting for a friend to arrive from California. I stood quietly watching them for a few minutes. It was not hard to figure out that they were playing Gin. I noticed a piece of paper in the man's trembling, wrinkled hand; the paper reminded me of the man holding it—tired and worn-looking, as though it had been folded and refolded many times. All that was on the paper were several columns of numbers. Every number except the very last number had a line drawn through it. This obviously is a scorecard, I thought to myself.

The man saw me watching them and smiled at me. Intrigued, I walked over, asking the man to explain the piece of paper to me.

"It's simple," he said. "My wife and I," he nodded at the petite, snow white-haired lady sitting next to him, "have been playing the same game of Gin for over 25 years. Our only rule is that we only play when we are in an airport."

"Who's winning?" I asked.

Pointing to his wife with a smile on his face, he said, "She is...by 40,000 points."

"40,000 points! Why do you keep playing with her?"

He shrugged his shoulders and, with a twinkle in his eye, he warmly replied, "What can I say? I love her."

I couldn't wait to call Gail and tell her that story. That's the kind of true story that we will cry over together. Playing Gin is as natural for Gail and me as drinking coffee. We've passed many hours together doing both.

Having to endure Parkinson's disease for almost half of my life, one of the most irritating of the side effects caused by the drugs necessary for normal functioning is dyskinesia. My dyskinesia is primarily in my right hand. It will occur at the most inopportune times. When it does occur, it's as if it has a mind of its own and demands total control It won't leave me alone to do something as simple as playing a game of cards. It commands attention even then.

Under normal circumstances, it takes two hands to play cards; two hands to shuffle the deck, two hands to deal the cards, two hands to put the cards in sequence in your hand. Usually, one hand is used to hold the cards, the other hand to draw and discard. These are all simple moves that most of us execute smoothly, without conscious thought of our actions. When, for whatever reason, one is unable to execute those moves fluidly, they become extremely complex and frustrating. If I didn't love to play cards, I would probably have thrown my hands up in defeat long ago.

Gail does all the shuffling, all the dealing, and keeps score. My only task is to hold on to my cards the best way I can, but if my hand doesn't want to be still, my cards are apt to go sailing across the room. Gail takes it all in stride. She jumps up and runs after them. There is no other way to respond other than to laugh about it.

"I don't mind running after your cards for you when they decide to take a flying leap. There's just one stipulation—we will not play cards in the wind!"

I shared the story with Gail about the Gin-playing Miami couple.

"If we had kept score all these years, too, how much would you think I'd be winning by?" I asked her teasingly.

"Oh, probably around 100,000 points," Gail replied.

"Why do you continue to play with me?"

With a slight shrug of her shoulders and a twinkle in her eyes, she said,

"What can I say—I love you!"

# *THAT SISTER THING*

That sister thing - If you have never had a sister then you won't know what in the world I'm talking about. A sister doesn't have to share a genetic bond with you. There is no course in school that you can take and graduate with a degree in sisterhood. With all the sophistication in stem cell research and brain mapping, I haven't heard of the possibility of implantation of a sister stem cell. For those of you who yearn for a sister, I wish there was such a thing for you. I'm sure those yearning for a sister have a mental checklist of the characteristics they think would make the best sister. Only those fortunate enough to belong to the sisterhood club know what those characteristics are. I am one of the fortunate ones.

The most important thing to know about sisterhood is that it is unexplainable. It is a deep-rooted mutual feeling of connectedness. Although it probably sounds corny, the best word I can think of to describe it is soul mates. The only sisterhood I am qualified to talk about is my own. I'm sure you could talk to 50 sisters and get 50 different definitions.

My sister knows my mind—what I think and what I know. My sister knows my heart—what I feel and what I love. My sister knows my soul—what I desire and what I strive for.

A few years ago, a good friend of mine, Mary Yost, also living with Parkinson's disease, lost her only sister and best friend to cancer.

Mary is the baby of her family. She doesn't know life without her sister. Her grief has been profound. Every time I think of her loss, my heart begins to hurt and I mourn for her, for me, and for all the sisters who are vulnerable to the inevitable death of their sister.

Within days of her sister's death, Mary was actively soliciting sisters. I volunteered. My own sister, Gail, volunteered, too. She's never met Mary. That's just how sacred sisterhood is.

I understand exactly how Mary feels. I am a baby sister. I don't know life without my sister. The thought of her not being here is overwhelming. Driving down the road one day, not very long ago, out of nowhere the thought of my sister dying filled my head. Almost immediately, my heart began to race; I couldn't catch my breath. I pulled the car over to the side of the road and waited for my breathing and heart rate to return to normal. What I really wanted to do then as well as now is to shout at the top of my lungs, "What will I do without you?" We live about 100 miles apart, but you know what? I think she would be able to hear me.

*I wrote the following letter just days after receiving a phone call from the wife of a good friend. Her husband, my friend Steve Mulligan, had just passed away. He was the first of my friends to die from complications of Parkinson's disease.*

## LETTER TO A FRIEND

Dear Steve,

You left us so suddenly, July 30, 1997. It takes me breath away to think about your being gone. I keep thinking that surely this is someone's idea of a bad joke. You were too young to die! You were only 49 years old. It seems like just yesterday that we last talked. I can still hear your soft, slow drawl. The drawl that always fooled me into thinking you were a good Southern boy, when in fact, you lived in Michigan. I remember our last conversation where I was giving you my usual cheerleader "rah " and you were making me giggle with that slow, dry wit of yours.

Until your death, I would become indignant when I overheard someone speak of another's death as being "from" Parkinson's disease. My curt reply was always, "We don't die from Parkinson's disease. We just sometimes wish we could." Now I am indignant because your death forces me to face the reality that Parkinson's disease does kill. For some, it's an emotional death; for others, it's a spiritual death. For you, my good friend, it was the ultimate, physical death.

I am angry at the stupid disease because it defeated you in your battle to survive. You, who were so gifted, so uniquely alive, so in love with life and always so full of hope; you had so much work left to do. We had many projects to work on together—The Mulligan Foundation, support groups, websites, just to name a few. We schemed and we dreamed with so many ideas and plans. The only thing we lacked was the time to implement them. You left too soon.

I am grateful for the time your Pallidotomy afforded you, but it wasn't enough and it wasn't soon enough, was it? The recent breakthroughs in medications and the Deep Brain Stimulation, to name a couple, didn't come in time for you.

Why is it that our very existence and the quality of our lives boil down to money? I hate that. I know that if scientific research had been adequately funded, you wouldn't have suffered as you did. Perhaps you would still be here today. Researchers keep taunting us with the possibility of a cure within my lifetime. These same people promised a cure within your lifetime, too. I honestly believe the cure is "just around the corner." The amount of money needed to take researchers around the corner is staggering, though.

For years, I closed my ears to the pleas to raise money for research. I am an old cheerleader with a social worker mentality. What do I know about fundraising? Your death forced me to think about the lack of funding from a very personal point of view. The financial issue becomes much more personal when, because of the disparity, someone I love dies. Your death provides for me the understanding, the determination, and passion to raise money for research. I don't want to lose another friend to this monster we call a disease.

I want you to know that you did not suffer needlessly. It served a purpose for those you left behind. Your proud, fighting spirit lives on in me and in all of your family and friends who were privileged to share a part of your unique life. Thank you, Steve, for showing me how to live my life with dignity and purpose.

Missing you,
Terrie

# LIVING WITH PARKINSON'S DISEASE

Living with Parkinson's disease, from my personal experience, is quite an interesting journey. I have heard many "mother-in-law" jokes over the years. Although I do not have the same first hand experience with a mother-in-law that I do with Parkinson's disease, I can see the similarity. I do not mean to suggest that all mothers-in-law are the same nor are all cases of Parkinson's disease the same. I am speaking strictly from a personal, lifelong relationship with Parkinson's disease.

Living with it—Parkinson's disease, that is—is comparable to stories I hear of living in the same house with a mother-in-law, two strong, independent forces occupying the same space with each one striving for control.

In the early years of the relationship, there is much to learn about the other, uncharted waters, so to speak. There is politeness and consideration between the two with neither trying to dominate nor control the other. Perhaps this is because each considers the living arrangements to be temporary. Call it what you want—denial, naiveté, ignorance, unrealistic optimism—maybe a little of each. It's just a short visit. She'll go home soon. Parkinson's disease is just a temporary invasion.

Unless you are either a prophet or a fortune teller with great intuitive powers, there's no way you can accurately predict the future... whether it is a mother-in law who neglected to tell you that she has made your home her permanent address or Parkinson's disease, which has also settled in for the long haul.

I must admit that I don't personally have much experience with mothers-in-law. I have only had one mother-in-law, and that seems like a lifetime ago, long before I had even uttered the words, Parkinson's disease. I lived 700 miles away from my mother-in-law, and I never knew her well. Well, except for the annual visit she would make to my house for the week that felt like eternity. My experience with Parkinson's disease is entirely different. It dropped in for what I presumed to be a visit when I was 28 years old. Unlike my mother-in-law, who, did go home after a week, I discovered 24 years after the initial visit from Parkinson's disease that IT'S STILL HERE! I must have learned a few tricks to help me cope with an unwanted houseguest who long ago outstayed its welcome. Otherwise, by now, surely I would be either dead or insane!

I learned early on with this disease the value of plastic. Plastic doesn't break—well, most of it doesn't. It just bounces when it falls. I should know. Living with unannounced, spontaneous bouts of involuntary movement (dyskinesia) in my right hand, I never know when an object is going to suddenly go flying out of my hand and shatter on the other side of the room. It usually happens when I am holding something very fragile, very expensive, or very hot. I long ago gave up on having a matched set of coffee mugs. I'm thinking seriously about going to a restaurant supply house and buying a case of "diner strength" white china. They are sturdy enough to withstand most minor accidents. In the case of a wild, uncontrollable movement, when I have flung a steaming, hot cup of coffee across the kitchen to shatter into small shards of china, it won't be a major loss. I'll simply pick up the broken pieces, throw them away, go to my reserve stock, replace the cup, let the dog lick up the spilt coffee, and I will still have a matching set of cups.

I used to have fantasies of taking up photography as a serious hobby. A few years ago, I invested in a nice 35mm camera. I lost it at a Parkinson's disease conference in Washington, D.C. I invested in a second 35mm camera. Someone stole if from my suitcase somewhere in route between the Philadelphia airport and the Atlanta airport. After much deliberation, I bought one more camera. One beautiful fall day, about 8 years ago, while living in Roanoke, Virginia, I decided to spend the day taking pictures of the beautiful foliage on the Blue Ridge Parkway. I was standing at the highest elevation on the parkway, at the peak of the "turning of the leaves" looking down at the valley below. *What a spectacular shot,* I thought to myself. I raised the camera to my eye, ready to snap the picture, when unexpectedly came that same violent burst of involuntary movement in my right hand. In the time that it takes for a camera shutter to blink, the fingers on my right hand, tightly gripping the camera, suddenly jerked open to a rigid position. My camera went sailing off that mountain way down into the valley below.

*Well,* I thought to myself, *there goes my future as a famous photographer.* Now, I leave photography to people whose hand movements are a bit more predictable than mine are.

My daily dependency on my Parkinson's disease medication, particularly Sinemet, is so strong that I would have an anxiety attack if I thought I was running low and wouldn't be able to get to the pharmacy for my refill. I rarely ever let my supply fall lower than a week's supply. My attitude changed dramatically once I learned how to go "carpet farming." When I find that my supply is low, I simply get down on my hands and knees and begin to comb through the carpet with my fingers searching for those stray blue, football-shaped pills that I am constantly dropping. The first and most obvious place I look is the floor on my side of the bed, as well as under the bed. I then progress to the living room where I search my recliner and the floor surrounding it. If I still haven't found enough to keep me going for a while, I check the pockets of my bathrobe, jeans, shorts, crevices in my purse and finally, my car. A normal daily supply of Sinemet for me is 10–12 pills, as I take one every two hours, around the clock. The last time I went "carpet farming," I found 60 pills, a five-day supply!

No one asks for a certain disease, at least, no one I know. When I was diagnosed with Parkinson's disease after four years of searching and finally admitting to myself that living in denial wasn't going to make it go away -only then did I figure out that if I wanted to survive this "nightmare" of a disease, I had better develop a keen sense of humor and quit taking myself so seriously. It has taken quite a few years, much hard work, and the love of a supportive and patient husband to help me see the humor in my daily life.

The next time you're on your hands and knees cleaning up the remains of the hot cup of coffee you just flung across the room, just tell yourself you really needed the exercise anyway. While you're down there, do a little carpet farming. You'll be surprised at what you will find.

# MUSINGS, OBSERVATIONS, AND OTHER UNSOLICITED OPINIONS

Let me preface this chapter by saying that very little of what I am about to discuss has any scientific data to back it up. These are simply personal thoughts and observations I have developed over the years that I have had Parkinson's disease and worked with others who are afflicted by it. It is my hope that these observations will lead others: patients, caregivers, doctors, and researchers—to pay closer attention to the subtleties of the disease. If this is done, I am sure quality of life and functionality will be enhanced. Often the subtleties make the difference.

Through my travels and my work at Emory University, I have encountered thousands of people with Parkinson's disease. I have empathized with them over the telephone; counseled them in the clinic; held their hands during surgery; visited in their homes; spoken with them and to them at their support groups; lobbied with and for them in Congress; walked together in Central Park; socialized in groups at parties; cried with them in hospitals, and prayed with and for them in churches. I have traveled from Florida to New York, from New Jersey to California, and from Washington State to Mexico on behalf of Parkinson's disease. During my travels, I have counted, analyzed, and questioned individuals and groups along the way. I have noticed several patterns that seem to be a little more than coincidence.

I read somewhere that left-handed people comprise approximately 10% of the general population. Being left-handed, this is naturally of interest to me. I began to look closely at the groups of Parkinson's patients across the country and found that 20-30% are left-handed. Have any studies been done in this area? I wonder.

79

While I was working with the Pallidotomy program at Emory University, I discovered the Pallidotomy roster consisted of three times as many men as women. Why? Are men greater risk takers than women when it comes to brain surgery? Do men have more severe cases of Parkinson's disease than women? Or is it that men are three times more likely to develop Parkinson's disease?

Studies have been done to compare the incidence rate of Parkinson's disease in the African American population to that of Caucasians. The study concluded no significant difference. A friend of mine, nurse coordinator for Emory's Movement Disorder Program, grew up in the very same rural area of Mississippi where the more than thirty-year-old study was conducted. She, coincidentally, is African American and agrees with me that, of the Parkinson's patients we have encountered, it is more likely 50 to 1 Caucasian. I worked with more than 100 people with Parkinson's disease in Washington, D.C. while lobbying for the passage of the Morris K. Udall Bill. In the four years I worked in that area, I met one African American with Parkinson's disease.

After many years of observing people with Parkinson's disease, I have concluded that there is a Parkinson personality. (Well, at least several common personality traits.) I once asked a well-known neuro-psychiatrist if he thought there were any common personality traits among PWP, (People with Parkinson's). In a word, he summed it up, in the men, particularly, narcissism. He said that women share the trait, too, but it was present more in men. Therefore, I have come up with my description of a typical Parkinson patient (certainly not to be taken for fact, but it does make one go "hmmm").

A typical Parkinson patient would be a left-handed, narcissistic, over-achieving, above-average in intelligence, articulate, creative, depressed male.

It is a fact that at least 50% of those diagnosed with Parkinson's also exhibit symptoms of depression and that depression, often, is the first symptom to appear. This does not mean that if one is depressed, one will develop Parkinson's disease.

One of my first memories following my Pallidotomy in 1993 was that of intense euphoria. The depression that I had experienced for years seemed to be gone. Over time, it became clear that the euphoria more resembled the manic phase of manic depression or bipolar disorder. I had never experienced this prior to surgery. Many, many people who underwent the same procedure also admitted to the same sensation. Is it possible that manic depression can be surgically induced?

I have noticed over the years that everything—and let me emphasize EVERYTHING—in my life affects my functional level. Something as seemingly trivial as constipation makes my symptoms worse. Equally trivial, it would seem, is a urinary tract infection. Let me give you an example:

About a year after my Pallidotomy, while I was still reaping near-normal benefits of the surgery, without warning, my Parkinson medication simply quit working. It was a Friday afternoon when I first noticed that my Parkinson symptoms were back in full force. There was no major event going on in my life at the time to warrant an emotional trigger for my symptoms to worsen suddenly. I did not feel physically ill, nor could I attribute it to any other factor. By Saturday afternoon, With Parkinson symptoms still full-blown, and no positive effect from the medication, I began to be alarmed. Not knowing what else to do, I called Dr. Vitek at home. He, too, became alarmed. I spent the next 24 hours in numerous telephone conversations with Drs. Vitek, DeLong, Watts, and Bakay. This was new territory for them, too. They had never encountered a situation where a Pallidotomy patient experienced such a dramatic change in functional level in such a short period for no explainable reason. By Sunday afternoon, the consensus was for me to drive to Atlanta and admit myself to Emory so they could monitor my condition and perform any necessary tests.

The first and foremost concern of the doctors' was that I had a brain shift or a brain injury. A MRI was ordered to determine if there had been any structural changes in my brain.

When those results came back normal, I had a complete urine and blood analysis. Tuesday, the 5th day of this ordeal, corresponded with the results of the blood work. I woke up that morning with the first signs of a UTI. The blood work confirmed it. The remarkable thing was that once the symptoms of the UTI appeared, my Parkinson medications suddenly began to work again. What a surprise for the doctors and me! Since then, I continue to have a UTI about once a year. Typically, I don't know immediately that I have an infection. The physical symptoms don't usually occur until the second or third day of poor response to medication. I have since learned that my body reacts in a similar fashion with any type of infection.

Since that first experience, I have tried to pay closer attention to the events and circumstances of my everyday life and how they affect my functional level. Here are some of the things I have observed.

Eating a large meal slows down the absorption of my medication, thereby causing a poor response to medication. Eating protein significantly slows down the absorption of medication, too. Any form of exercise depletes my dopamine level. Any change in barometric pressure is sure to affect my functional level. Any change in emotion: sadness, excitement, anger, fear, or depression—causes me to be less responsive to my medication. The same is true for fatigue.

If the situation is acute yet temporary, then my functional decline is also temporary. If, however, one or more factors is chronic or long-lasting, then my functional level is similarly affected. I hope that some of these observations will benefit other people, as well as give insight to their doctors.

# KILL THE POSSUM

Recently, I returned home from running errands to find unwelcome guests in my house. I unlocked the front door and walked into the living room. Out of the corner of my eye, to my right, in the kitchen, under the kitchen table, I spied what initially looked like two giant wharf rats. I immediately let out a bloodcurdling scream and quickly backed out of the front door, slamming it as I exited. My heart was pounding as hard and loud as a stampede of elephants.

*"What were those critters?"* I wondered, as I slowly got my breath back. Obviously, I am not very brave when it comes to finding my home invaded by unwelcome four-legged guests of any kind. I slowly tiptoed up to the kitchen window, stood up on my tiptoes, and hesitantly peered in the window. There they were, under the kitchen table still, one light gray one and a brown one. As I watched through the window, the brown one scampered across the floor towards the refrigerator. *Oh, this is just great*, I thought, *Now they have split up*. But, as I watched the one running across the floor, I was able to get a clear look at him. They weren't rats after all. They were baby possums! How did they get inside my house?

John and I both knew that we had an adult possum living under our house. We have heard it on numerous occasions under the office floor. We first saw it one evening in June about two years ago, as he came from under the house and sauntered toward the woods. I have seen plenty of possums in my life, but until then they had all been dead, roadkill along the side of the highway. This was my first introduction to live possums. It was not a pleasant sight!

John has tried to kill this possum for the two years it has been living with us. He was successful in shooting the possum only once. All he accomplished was to make the possum angry. In the excitement of seeing the possum, running to find the gun before he got away and actually hitting him with the bullets, John discovered that what he had shot it with was snake shot. Sometime earlier, he had loaded the clip with three snake shot before the hollow points. Oh, he hit the possum all three times. Each time he hit the possum, it would stop its leisurely saunter into the woods, turn around, and stare at John with those dark little beady eyes as if to say, "STUPID!" By the time he had gone through the three rounds of snake shot and finally got to the hollow points, the gun jammed, it was dark outside, and the possum was in the woods. So much for possum hunting.

We didn't know the possum was a female. I, at least, didn't know it, even though, on several occasions, we had heard what sounded like the possum entertaining another possum of the opposite sex under the office.

Therefore, when I saw the baby possums under my kitchen table, although I didn't know how they'd gotten there, I did know where they'd come from. I knew one thing. I was not going back into that house until somebody came and got those possums out of my kitchen.

I was hysterical, laughing and crying at the same time. I called John, at work, on the cell phone.

"John, there are two baby possums in the kitchen, under the kitchen table."

"How did they get there?" he calmly asked.

"How the hell should I know?" I screamed hysterically.

"Well, what do you want me to do about it? I'm at work, thirty minutes away."

"I don't know," I sobbed.

"Do you want me to come home early?"

Again, I said, "I don't know."

There were a couple of minutes of silence.

Finally, John said, "I'll be home in just a little bit."

I breathed a sigh of relief. I was thinking to myself, though, as I hung up the telephone, how many times do I call my husband at work? Almost never! How many times do I call him at work with hysteria in my voice? Even rarer than almost never! Moreover, he had to ask if I wanted him to come home early. Duh! If I had just wanted to call someone and chat about the damn invasion of my home by hideous baby varmints, I could just as well have called my sister, who lives 120 miles away! She was too far away to save me, but she would have had me laughing about them before I hung up.

That day was one that I had to pick up my nephew, B.J., from school. I looked at the clock in the car. It was 3:30. I knew I had to hurry or I would be late. In all the excitement, I had to go to the bathroom very badly. I wasn't about to go back in my house to go to the bathroom. No way, no how! I got in my car and drove over to B.J.'s house, which was on the way to the school. Thank goodness, Julie, my sister-in-law, never locks her doors. I ran to the bathroom, getting there just in time before wetting my pants! Having gotten that out of the way, I hurriedly drove to pick B.J. up from school.

I was the last car to get to the school and B.J., the only student left, was pacing up and down the walkway. B.J., thirteen at the time, was at the ravenous time in his life—always hungry; I knew he might not survive the trip home from school without food to sustain him. If you have ever had a thirteen-year-old boy, you know exactly what I'm talking about. The foods he loves more than anything are fresh fruits. It has become a ritual with us that whenever I pick him up from school, I always have fresh fruit in the car ready to eat. On this day, however, there was no fruit. The bananas were in the kitchen with the possums.

I was curious to see whether B.J. would mention the fruit, or rather, the absence of fruit. He got in the car, spoke to me, and then started looking around the car. I waited a few seconds. He didn't mention it. I should have known that he had better manners than that!

"Do you want to know why I didn't bring fruit with me today?" I asked.

"Yeah," said B.J. "I'm starving."

"There are two baby possums in my kitchen," I said, "and I was afraid to go back in the house to get it."

B.J. didn't crack a smile. He sat there and studied me for a minute. Finally, in a slow, serious voice, he said, "I hope they don't eat my fruit."

Within just a few minutes, we were back at my house. I made B.J. go in the house ahead of me to scout out the possums and give an "all clear" sign before I would even walk inside. I cautiously walked into the house, looking around me with every step I took, just knowing, any second, possums were going to come out of hiding and scare the hell out of me. I made it to the recliner without incident while B.J. went to the kitchen to make sure his fruit was safe.

I was sitting there, for maybe five minutes, thinking to myself that I might have to stay in the recliner until Johnny came home from work. It was then that I heard his car in the driveway. He *had* heard the hysteria in my voice! He *had* figured out what a dumb question he had asked me!

As he came through the front door, he was struggling to keep the smile off his face and the laughter out of his voice as he asked me the whereabouts of our unwanted houseguests.

"How the heck do I know? The last time I saw them they were both in the kitchen."

"You mean you didn't keep them cornered where you could see them until I got home?" he asked.

I couldn't very well keep the possums cornered and pick B.J. up from school at the same time, now, could I? I'm going to give him an excuse and say that he forgot about the part where I had to leave to go get B.J. because no husband in his right mind would ask his already hysterical wife that question otherwise. Therefore, I just looked at him—hard—giving him one of those "mama" looks, and said nothing.

B.J. found his fruit, unharmed, and sat in the living room with me eating a banana while Johnny went possum hunting through the house. A few minutes later, I saw Johnny crouched in a low, bent position, tiptoeing through the living room, his finger to his lips, whispering in his "Elmer Fudd" voice, "Shhh! Be vewy, vewy quiet; I am hunting possum."

With the same deadpan face and flat, emotionless voice, I could hear B.J. softly singing, "Kill the possums."

Johnny and B.J. searched the house over and did not see any evidence of our home invaders. We spent the rest of the evening uneventfully and went to bed, as usual.

I woke up at five o'clock the next morning feeling something tickling my arm. I opened my eyes and found myself staring into the small, dark beady eyes of one of the baby possums tickling my arm with his nose. Johnny woke up at five o'clock to the sound of a blood-curdling scream and opened his eyes to see his wife, me, catapulting across the bed, in mid-air, to land on top of him.

"There's a possum in the bed with us!" I screamed.

Johnny, trying to soothe me while at the same time totally not believing me, gently suggested that I might have been dreaming.

"I was not dreaming!" I sobbed. "I know what I saw. I opened my eyes and found myself looking into the eyes of one of those possums. He was tickling my arm with his nose!"

"Well, where did he go?" Johnny asked.

For the second time in 24 hours, I screamed, "How the heck do I know? Find the dad-gum thing and kill it!"

Just to humor me, I found out later, Johnny got out of bed with nothing on but a t-shirt and grabbed a piece of plastic PVC pipe and walked through the house, knowing in his mind that he wasn't going to find anything. And he didn't. While he was gone, I cautiously slid from the bed to the recliner, which was positioned about two feet from the foot of my side of the bed. I huddled in the chair with my arms wrapped around my legs, shaking all over. In a few minutes, Johnny came back in the bedroom and announced that he could not find anything. He laid the PVC pipe on the counter in the kitchen before coming into the bedroom. I could not believe what happened next! My wonderful husband got back in the bed, pulled the covers up around him, turned over, and was going back to sleep!

I was still huddled in the recliner, shaking like a leaf, a multitude of thoughts bombarding my mind all at once. *How can he go back to sleep while I'm sitting over here, clearly, still in a crisis? He doesn't believe me! He thinks I'm hallucinating!* Oh, Lord, I prayed, *if I truly am hallucinating just go ahead and take me now. If I'm not hallucinating, show me the possum now or Johnny will never believe anything I say to him.*

At about that time, I was staring at the bed when I noticed a throw pillow at the foot of the bed moving up and down. I sat quietly, not breathing, just watching it for a minute, thinking, if I tell Johnny there's a pillow moving on its own, he'll think I've lost my mind! Again, I let out a blood-curdling scream. Johnny sat back up in bed.

"What now?" he asked wearily.

"There's something under that pillow," I said, as I pointed to the throw pillow. Or, at least, I think I pointed to it.

"What pillow?" Johnny started throwing all the pillows around, again seeing nothing. As I continue staring, I saw the covers on the corner of the bed begin to move. I continued screaming and pointing, trying to think of the word for cover or blanket, comforter, anything. All I could do, though, was point and stutter. After what seemed like an eternity, Johnny moved the covers away from the corner of the bed and saw the baby possum an inch away from his hand. He said to me, "Keep your eye on him."

Like I was going somewhere?

He ran to the kitchen, got the PVC pipe, and came back to the bedroom. The next words out of his mouth were, "Are you ready for this?"

The following sequence of events seemed to take place in slow motion. Johnny pulled the PVC pipe/club back over his shoulder into the first stance of a golf swing, followed through by smacking the possum, sending him flying off the bed. His follow through ended when the PVC pipe encountered the lower part of my right leg. The result of the golf swing was one dead possum and a bump on my leg the size of a golf ball.

When Johnny realized what he had done he asked, "Why didn't you move?"

"Duh, I have Parkinson's disease. I can't exactly move that fast on command."

Then came the final question, the question that I unequivocally rank as the number one dumbest questions my otherwise intelligent husband has ever asked me.

"Baby, did it look like one of the possums you saw earlier?" Like my son, Matthew, told me later, I guess I should have named them so I would recognize them in a lineup.

It's been a while now since the possum invasion. I still look under the kitchen table every time I walk into my house. The knot on my leg is just a memory. Whenever I see B.J., he still sings softly, "Kill the possum." Most important, though, according to my golf club/PVC pipe-swinging husband, is the moral of this story: "If your wife ever wakes you up at 5:00 in the morning screaming, 'there's a possum in the bed,' whatever you do, DON'T TEE HER OFF!"

# BEATRICE FLORENCE

The very best part of summer vacation, actually any time I had time out of school, was going to Macon to stay with Grandma. She was the light of my life and I, in return, was the light of her life. While I have never been completely confident about many things in my life, the one thing I have never doubted was Grandma's unconditional love for me. She was a safe, warm haven whenever I needed one. I can't even think about her for more than a minute without my eyes filling with tears and my heart beginning to hurt.

Oh Lord, how I miss her! She left too soon! I never had the chance to know her or for her to know me when I became a grown-up. I never had the chance to watch her enjoy and love my children and to think that they are as wonderful as I think they are. I was sixteen when she died. She was sixty-two. Thirty-five years she has been gone from my life, but, oh, the memories I have of her! The memories never go away. Neither do the dreams.

Beatrice Kennington Dorman was born one of ten children in the rural middle part of Georgia in Twiggs County. She didn't have a middle name. She said the reason she didn't was because she was born into a poor family and her parents couldn't afford middle names for all the children. Therefore, the girls—Gladys, Pauline, Mary, Beatrice, and Claude—were given just one name. The boys, however, were given two fine, distinguished names— John Homer, Garner Mercer, Jerome Pinkney, Henry Grady, and Leon Kennington. Grandma always wanted a middle name so one day she decided to give herself one. It was Florence. She thought Florence was the most beautiful name in the world. She, therefore, from that day forward, in her imagination and in her play with me, became Beatrice Florence Kennington Dorman.

I don't know for fact but rumor has it that Grandma's daddy was a mean, abusive man. That would explain why she married a mean, abusive man, I guess. That would be my granddaddy Dorman, Earlie Dorman. They ran away to get married when Grandma was nineteen years old. Granddaddy was twenty-five. They eloped one night in June on Granddaddy's big ole Indian motorcycle. Granddaddy drove with Grandma sitting next to him in the sidecar. They were both dressed fit to kill in their fine, leather-riding outfits; leather helmets, goggles, gloves, leather jacket, leather jodhpurs, and leather-riding boots. I'm telling you what, Grandma was a woman before her time! She had short, bobbed hair, stylish for the time. Pictures are the only place I have seen her with anything but grayish white hair. When she was young, though, it was a beautiful dark brown.

Granddaddy's folks came from Alabama, so that is where they eloped to—the courthouse in Phoenix City, Alabama. Phoenix City is really just over the state line, right next to Columbus, GA.

Granddaddy took Grandma back home that night after they got married. She got a spanking from her daddy for getting home late! They kept their marriage a secret for a month until Grandma gathered up the courage to tell her daddy. She knew that her parents did not like Granddaddy, and they thought she married beneath herself. I think I agree with them. I just think Grandma was so unhappy at home that she would have married just about anyone to get away. Earlie Dorman, six years older, was just the first one to come along.

They were quite a pair—Mutt and Jeff? Granddaddy was 6'7" to Grandma's 5'2". Oh, the memories I have of her; the softness of her skin when she hugged me; her silky white hair, so fine and soft, yet so thick; sitting in her lap brushing and playing with her hair until I grew tired of it; lying across her lap, drifting off to sleep to the lull of her soft voice gossiping with the neighbor and her fingernails softly scratching circles on my back. No one has ever been able to soothe me like that since Grandma.

The memories roar in so fast they seem to stumble on each other. I strive to keep up with them but can't type the words fast enough before another one crashes in. The healthy, active

Grandma who would take me to run errands with her. Just for fun, she would drive the old '54 roadster that Granddaddy built the year I was born. He built it for his 6'7" frame so it was comical to see Grandma with a big pillow behind her back so she could sit close enough to reach the steering wheel, gas, and brake pedals. She was tough, though and wasn't a bit afraid to drive that monster of a car. We were a sight; I'd imagine, pulling into the parking lot of Ethridge's, the local meat market where she shopped. They all knew me there. The first stop was to the meat counter in the back where Mr. Ethridge would give me a raw hot dog to eat while we shopped, on the house, of course.

I remember the playful, carefree, creative Grandma who sang made up, nonsensical songs while we rode down the roads. I can't even remember the words now. I do remember the words to *The Headless Horseman*, a poem that I loved to hear her recite.

I remember the risqué Grandma that only wore underwear to church on Sundays. I remember those housedresses that she always wore. They had flowers on them, two pockets in the front and snaps instead of buttons. She probably had a different one for every day of the week. In the winter, she'd stand in the hall, straddling the floor furnace, the hot air causing her dress to billow up around her. Suddenly I could hear her poot. Each time she pooted, she'd let out a sigh of relief. She was so funny to watch. She had a wicked sense of humor and loved to tease.

I remember the happy-go-lucky Grandma that would dance around the house barefoot, playing *Home on the Range* on her harmonica, the gentle, patient Grandma who always answered my questions and never seemed to tire of my incessant chatter, the compassionate and deeply spiritual Grandma, who was firmly anchored in her steadfast devotion to God, who never missed a Sunday in church, and who fed and clothed strangers who knocked on her door and gave them her last dollar because she figured they needed it worse than she did.

I remember the loyal Grandma, who stuck by Granddaddy's side through thick and thin, neglect and abuse, and never said a word! The politically minded and socially savvy Grandma, who organized political campaigns and March of Dime drives and worked at them tirelessly because she cared about and felt a responsibility to do her part to make this world a better place to live.

I remember the practical yet impatient Grandma, who would save us all from having to sing 20 verses of *Just as I Am* at the dedication part of the Sunday church service. The preacher was not going to end the song until someone walked down that aisle and rededicated his life to Christ. Grandma had fried chicken warming in her oven at home. She knew the longer we sat there, the drier it would be when we finally ate it. Grandma began scanning the congregation during the first verse of the song looking for someone, anyone to walk down that aisle to the altar. If, by the second verse, no one got up, Grandma would do it. We all counted on Grandma to get us home before the chicken dried out. I suspect even the preacher was grateful to Grandma for helping him to end the service. She probably rededicated her life to Christ at least once a month.

Grandma, you left us too soon. You gave so much and meant so much and were loved so much by so many. You left when I needed you the most. You were my best friend, my playmate, my cheerleader, my hero, You were a mother to me.

# *MY STARR IN THE EAST*

My first marriage took place when I was a mere nineteen. My divorce occurred when I was a nearly mere twenty-nine. I had brain surgery for the first time, to relieve symptoms of Parkinson's disease, at thirty-nine. There is something about the number nine.

Soon after my divorce, I was certain that I would marry again. All I needed was to find the right man. How hard could that be? After a couple of years, I somewhat just gave up and became very cynical. Whenever the subject of marriage came up, I would snidely remark, "If I am ever going to get married again, you know to look for a star in the East." It's true what "they" say. You'd better be careful what you wish for because you just might get it!

It started like this:

"Would you do me the honor of dancing with me? You look like you are having such a good time."

That was the beginning line to the best of my life.

The time was November 6, 1999. The event was my niece, Leigh's, wedding.

As he took me in his arms for the first slow dance of the evening, his strong hands pressed against the small of my back. Standing 6'1", he looked down into my inquisitive brown eyes with his dark hazel eyes.

"Hi. My name is John Starr, and I'm second cousin to the groom's father, Hylos the Elder, on his mother's side. The groom, Hylos III's grandmother, was my father's sister. Who are you and how are you related?"

"I am the bride's favorite aunt. My name is Terrie Willis-Whitling. Leigh's mother, Gail, is my sister."

That slow, low, Southern drawl, so sexy, so sultry—it had been too long since I had heard that familiar accent whispering what sounded like sweet, soulful music to my ear. I had almost forgotten the smoothness, the finesse, and, yes, the charm only a true-blooded Southern gentleman can exude with confidence. Boy was he exuding confidence! What a gentleman he was, too. His mama, Mae-Mae, too, would have been so proud of him.

"You are absolutely stunning!" he said, as he softly caressed me with his eyes.

I was stunning! Wearing my black velvet and satin dress with the slit that went from my ankle up to my thigh and off-the-shoulder bodice, I felt sexy for the first time in years, and I, too, exuded confidence.

It was a magical night, and I felt much like Cinderella with my prince by my side. What a sucker I am for beards and those dimples deepening as his smile broadened. My heart was melting.

Later that evening, we went outside to blow bubbles as Leigh and Hylos ran through the lines formed all the way to their waiting limo. A few minutes later, we were standing over to the side of the staircase leading up to the reception room. I suddenly felt like an Amazon in my platform sandals. Until that break, we had been dancing for over two hours. Johnny left my side only once.

"You are so beautiful. I am so taken with you. You are doing something to me, girl." When he was near me, his touch never left me. He left my side only once during that night; otherwise, never taking his eyes off me. I felt beautiful under his gentle, steady gaze.

He was so gentle and understanding before he even knew. On the other hand, did he? When my right hand began marching to its own beat, Johnny would simply fold my hand into his, give it a little squeeze, and say, "It's okay."

"I need for you to know that I have Parkinson's disease," I told him. "That is why my balance, rhythm, and timing are off. I used to teach aerobics. Those were the first things to go."

"Thank you for telling me. I knew when I first saw you that something was wrong. What first attracted me to you though was your spunk and pinash. The rest doesn't matter. It's just surface stuff. Then when we started talking, I was taken by your mind. Don't ever apologize for anything concerning your condition.

You didn't ask for it. You did nothing to deserve it. You have no control over it. Besides, it's just a part of you."

We went back outside at the break following Leigh and Hylos's departure. Ever the gentleman, he asked, "Will it bother you if I smoke?"

"It will only bother me if you don't offer me one," I said.

There was stone rectangular flower box on the sidewalk just next to where Johnny and I were standing while we smoked.

"I need to sit down for a minute, if you don't mind." Before he could reply, I had inched down until I was perched on the corner of the flower box. I kicked my shoes off and put my bare feet on the cool concrete. I pulled the skirt of my velvet dress snugly around my knees. Thinking I might be cold, Johnny wordlessly took his jacket off and slipped it around my bare shoulders.

"Have I told you how simply stunning you look tonight?" he asked.

Looking up at him, laughing, I said, "Yes, you have, but you can tell me again."

In the next second, Johnny asked, "Will you marry me?"

"No! Hell no! I have been married once and that was enough for me. I won't ever get married again."

"I just meant for the weekend."

I was still laughing when Karen, a friend of the groom's family, walked up to where we were standing. It was startling how much she resembled the actress Linda Dano.

"What's so funny?" she asked.

With a wounded look on his face, Johnny whined, "I just asked Terrie to marry me and she turned me down. She didn't just say no, she said Hell No! Not even for the weekend? I asked her. She won't even marry me for the weekend. I am crushed! After all, we have known each other for a grand total of 2 hours."

The disc jockey, hired for the reception, packed up his gear at midnight and headed home. I still felt like Cinderella at the ball, beautiful, elegant and yes, even stunning. I had never had so much fun in the town of my childhood. I wasn't ready for it to end. As if reading my mind, Johnny, said, "I don't want this night to end. I want to spend more time with you. Is there somewhere close by where we can get a drink?"

"There's a place just across the square there." I pointed over to Harper's Tavern. "I grew up next-door neighbors with the owner. I think they quit serving alcohol at midnight on Saturdays, though."

"Let's go, then," said Johnny.

Three of us, including Karen, the Linda Dano look-alike, started across the street and saw Hylos's brother, Robert, carrying a case of wine from the reception. Johnny said, "Do you mind?" as he grabbed a bottle out of the box. Robert didn't care. "It's paid for. Help yourself."

It was just after midnight on Sunday morning. Georgia's Blue Law prohibits the sale of alcohol after midnight on Saturday.

The bar was thick with smoke and brimming with people. As we entered the tavern, I warned Johnny that I would probably know the majority of the people there. As it turned out, I was right. I was on a first name basis with everyone there. Several others were as formally dressed as we were, having just left another wedding reception across town. Sam and Paula Goodrich, whom I have known for years, were among them. We were sitting at adjacent tables so began talking to each other. Eventually we began dancing, first by swapping off partners and ultimately dancing in a group. We danced until the band stopped playing at 2AM.

As the final song ended, we began saying our goodbyes. I hugged Paula and kissed Sam. Laughing hysterically, I watched while Johnny did the same thing. He hugged Paula and kissed Sam! Later he asked me, "Did I really kiss Sam before we left?"

"Yes," I said, "but at least you didn't kiss him on the mouth. You grabbed his face in your hands and kissed him on the cheek."

"I wonder how weird he thought I was," Johnny mused.

"Actually, it looked to me like he thought it was pretty funny."

Even then, I knew there was an attraction to Johnny that was different from other "first dates." I couldn't describe it, but whatever it was, I didn't want it to end. I also knew that Johnny felt the same way. Of course, I might have known that because he said, maybe a dozen times that night, "I've had SUCH a good time tonight."

It was after 4 AM when I dropped Johnny off at the motel. "When will I see you again? When are you coming to see me in Batesburg? I want to see you again."

"So do I," I sighed. "I have to go back home to Roanoke tomorrow."

"Well, why don't you stop in Batesburg on your way home? We can spend more time together. I really want to get to know you better."

"I don't go through South Carolina," I said.

"Well, you could. It wouldn't be out of your way. We need to spend some time together. I had so much fun with you that I don't want it to end."

Johnny was being so honest, so open with his feelings. I felt very flattered. It had been a long time since a man had said the kind of things Johnny said to me. I knew that I didn't want this to end either. Was it possible that this was more than just a good time for one night? Even though I was feeling the same things he was expressing to me, I was afraid to show it. I was shy and more than a little hesitant to show my emotions this early. I wanted to be more cautious with my words.

"I had a great time, too, and I want to get to know you better, too. Since I'm leaving for Roanoke later today, do you want to ride with me? I could drop you off in Batesburg.

"That's a good idea. I'd love to ride with you. Since I rode here with my sister, I need to check with her and be sure she doesn't have a problem with it. My daddy always told me, 'Always go home from the party with the one that you came with.' Why don't I call you later this morning after I talk to her?"

He did call later that morning. but I missed it. I saw on mama's caller ID that he had called, so I tried to call him back at the motel. He didn't answer. Oh no, don't tell me I missed him! I looked at the clock and saw that it was 8:30. Surely, he had not left already! I went to sleep thinking about him, woke up thinking about him, and now could think of nothing but him! *Oh hell,* I thought to myself. *What do I have to lose?* I hurriedly finished dressing, grabbed my car keys, and ran to find him. I hoped I wasn't too late. What excuse could I use for just showing up at his motel unannounced? Looking down at the passenger's seat to where he sat last night, I spied his tie. He had left it in the car last night. Perfect! A legitimate mission was now at hand—to deliver the tie to its rightful owner. Yeah, right. I know it was a flimsy excuse, but it was the best I could do under the circumstances. Besides, it would save me humiliation if he decided against riding home with me.

I remembered him telling me his room number last night. I felt like an idiot knocking on his door at 9:00 in the morning. No one answered. Now I really had a sinking feeling in the pit of my stomach that I had just missed him. I decided, as a last ditch effort, to walk around the motel. Maybe he was visiting in a relative's room or outside somewhere talking.

Wow! There he was! My heart pounding, I walked over to where he was playing ball with his nephews. When he looked up, he had the most beautiful smile on his face. He said, "Oh good, I was afraid I'd missed you!"

I felt like a teenager again, nervous, giddy, butterflies in my stomach. Not knowing what to say, I held up his tie. "You forgot something." After a couple of minutes of meaningless banter, I cut to the chase and boldly asked, "Would you still like for me to give you a ride home?"

"Yes," he said, "I'd love to spend the day with you. I haven't said anything to my sister, Julie, though. I wasn't sure if you would change your mind. Give me a few minutes to get my things and be sure she's okay with it."

I nodded and said, "I'll wait for you in the car. It's parked right across from your room."

Less than five minutes later, John was in the car with me ready to begin our day together. What a day it was, too!—an unseasonably warm day filled with sunshine and laughter with the first man that could make me laugh, cry, and wet my pants all at the same time.

It would have been so easy to stay there in Batesburg with him. Everything just seemed so right! I wasn't ready to admit to myself that I was already falling in love with this man who lived two states away from me.

After that weekend, we spent countless hours on the telephone, every single day! Hours of laughing, crying, telling jokes, using four syllable words. A week passed until I could see him again. It seems like months. Johnny came to Roanoke the next weekend. We had so much fun. I have never felt so at peace, so at home, as comfortable with anyone as I did with John.

I KNEW by the time he left Sunday night. I whispered softly in his ear, "I love you, Johnny."

"How much do you love me, Baby girl?"

"I love you enough to marry you."

"I love you forever and ever," he said.

I watched from my second floor apartment as the love of my life walked to his car below. Sensing that I was looking down at him, he looked up from where he stood in the middle of the street and yelled, "I love you, Baby girl!"

Now what? I wondered. My obligations continued in New Jersey. I had promised to be there for Thanksgiving. I sure wasn't looking forward to going, but I couldn't let Jean, Rol, Kymmy, and Gretchen down. They were depending on me. I was back in the stressful yet familiar surroundings of caring for Rol—scurrying to get Christmas ready for his two girls. I was simply going through the motions though. My heart wasn't in it. My heart was in Batesburg, South Carolina with John Bernie Starr. Why did I feel so sad? So alone? Even though I was around many people, none of them was named John Bernie Starr. As if a bolt of lightening hit me, I knew I was in the wrong place!

"Come home, Baby Girl."

I ran like hell.

"Welcome home, Baby Girl."

Home, at last.

January 2, 2000, 4 PM

"I, Terrie, take you Johnny, to be my husband, secure in the knowledge that you will be my constant friend, my faithful partner in life, and my one true love. On this special day, I give to you, in the presence of God and our family and friends, my promise to stay by your side as your faithful wife in sickness and health, joy and sorrow, the good times as well as the bad. I promise to love you without reservation, comfort you in times of distress, and encourage you to achieve all of your goals. Laugh with you, cry with you, and grow with you in mind and spirit, always to be open and honest with you and cherish you as long as we both shall live."

I always wanted to be a star. I found a Starr in the East, in Batesburg, South Carolina.

I am a Starr.

# *TURNING 50*

When I first started writing this piece, I was on the verge of turning 50. That seemed like such a mystical number, an age that has never seemed quite real for me. It always sounded old to me until I turned 49. It still sounds old for everybody else. For me, though, well I might as well be 24 or 42 because there is no age that feels right when I try it on. Do I look 50? I look in the mirror trying to figure out how one knows what 50 looks like. I don't think I look 50. I don't feel 50. But I don't feel 30 either. Teenage boys and twenty-somethings' still give me a second look when sitting next to me at a red light (okay, once!). Truck drivers still try to flirt with me on the interstate (occasionally).

I still don't wear a bra or panties or pantyhose or makeup. I do still wear tee shirts, blue jeans, and overalls. I still love to play games, say ugly words, have slut days and sleep in the nude. I still think about sex a lot and still like it. Maybe 50 looks different in different parts of the country. I'm a Southern 50. Southern 50 women might be different from Northern 50 women or Midwestern 50 women.

In a way, I am glad it's taken me a while to write this piece about being 50. Now I have lived through it and can tell you that it is highly overrated! I believed everything Oprah said about turning 50 and was sure that it was gonna be an "Oprah year" for me; at the very least, a Jane Fonda year.

That is a big fat NO! If anything, it was the total opposite of what I expected. I would even go so far as to say that it was one of the worst years of my adult life. I gained 50 pounds. What was I thinking that I should mark the passage of time with 1 pound for every year of life? I didn't get in shape. I didn't finish writing this book. In fact, I didn't finish anything I started during the year. I didn't even finish reading a book.

Maybe I feel different because I never expected to live to be 50 and to experience what 50 feels and looks like. I've had Parkinson's disease for almost half my life. The only thing in my life that I have done longer than have Parkinson's disease is to be a mother. I have almost 30 years of motherhood under my belt. For the past 23 years, I thought one of three things would happen to me by the age of 50: I would either be dead from complications of Parkinson's disease, I would be dead from suicide over having PD, or I would be cured. None of these three things have happened. I just got fat! I'm still very much alive, I am now 52, and I have high hopes again. I am finally a grandmother! I am still married to the love of my life, a younger man—happily—oh, and I still have Parkinson's disease.

The only one of those things that seems like it might change anytime soon is the 52. I'm expecting to see 53 and 63 and maybe even 73. That's kind of a cool thought. I also still expect to have Parkinson's disease. Hey, I've kept it this long, why get rid of it now? I think the Republicans are going to see to it that research doesn't find a cure in my lifetime anyway. Maybe I can at least break the cycle of gaining a pound for every year I age. See, my goals are much simpler now, the older I get.

*I wrote this piece during the years I spent in Washington, D.C. advocating for an increase in funding for Parkinson's disease research.*

## CHAMPION

I want to say to the world, "Are you watching? Look closely. Don't shy away. Don't belittle or ridicule. Look closely because the next victim could be you."

I want to say to the world, "Are you listening? We need your help. We need you to walk for those of us who can no longer walk. We need you to speak on behalf of those of us who can no longer be heard. We need you to be our champion in the battle for public awareness of a disease that is crippling an important segment of our working population—the thousands of young to middle-aged Americans disabled by Parkinson's disease.

"We need for you to become our champion because the next victim could be you. If it isn't enough that you be a champion of your peers, also know that the next victim could be your child."

Help us to dispel a myth! Parkinson's disease doesn't just afflict older citizens. It happened to me at twenty-eight. It caught many of my friends off guard at—four, eighteen, twenty-six, thirty-two, forty—etc. Help us, with your compassion and understanding, to have the confidence to come forward, shirking our security of invisibility, to bravely show ourselves to others. Walk by our sides as we show society that underneath the masked, expressionless faces, the unintelligible speech, the slow shuffling, shaking gait lurk bright, intelligent, creative, sensitive, loving mothers, fathers, sisters, brothers, and children—people no different from you in our desire to work, create, love, procreate, and live our lives with dignity. Help us to come off the sidelines of life with the opportunity to participate in life alongside you—richly, fully, and purposefully.

We are so often misunderstood! We need your help—not tomorrow, next week, or next year. We need your help now! We know all too well how precious life is. We want the same

103

opportunity as you to fully experience; to participate actively in the precious event we call LIFE.

I want to say to the world, "Are you listening? Can you hear me? Do you care?"

# *WHAT IF?*

It's interesting, to me, how the world events of the day can have such a profound effect on your thoughts and actions, even when that event did not affect you personally. Such is the case with me. If I seem to wander and ramble in my thoughts, try to bear with me because there is a point to all of it. I just can't start in the present day and have it make any sense. I think this is one of those times that God proves to me, one more time, as if I had any doubts, that everything that happens to us is by divine plan and has purpose.

I'm going to start forty years ago when I was just ten years old. I was "in love" for the first time. Well, maybe it was a ten-year-olds version of being in love, but it is as real to me today as it was forty years ago. There are some memories that time does not erase. Love is one of them. His name was Jimmy. It was the first day of school, and I was in Mrs. Cooke's 5th grade class.

Sandersville is a very small town, and going back to school usually meant being in the same room with the same people as the year before. When someone new moved to town, believe me, everyone noticed. In 1965, a new family moved to town—Jimmy Sr. and Sylvia, and the children: Jimmy, Jr., Bob, Charlotte, Linda, and little Ernie.

Jimmy, the oldest, was in my class in the 5th grade. When I first looked at him, I felt my heart skip a beat. He was so cute and so different looking from the rest of the boys my age, which I had known for most of our lives. He had blonde hair, with a longish Beatle haircut and beautiful blue eyes. Did I mention that he was cute? I don't remember specifics but at some point I let him know in my ten-year-old way that I liked him, and he let me know in his ten-year-old way that he liked me. I guess that we were "going together." That phrase used to drive both my dad and me crazy. I'd say, "I'm going with Jimmy." Daddy would say, "Where are you going with him?" I'd sigh and squeal, "NOWHERE! We're just going together."

I don't remember how long the romance lasted. About as long as most ten-year-old romances last I would guess—a week, a month, three months. It lasted long enough for me to give him British Sterling cologne for Christmas. It lasted long enough for me to remember wearing his ID bracelet with his name on it. That is how you knew if you were, "going with someone" or not, if they gave you their ID bracelet to wear. Of course, when you broke up, you had to give it back so he could give it to the next girl. Many girls wore Jimmy's bracelet in the 5$^{th}$ grade, but I'm sure I was the first.

We "went together" long enough to meet at the picture show on Friday nights and sit together during the movie. It wasn't long before we got caught, though, by my brother, Mark, who was eleven or twelve at the time, and hated girls. He sneaked up behind us in the theater and caught us holding hands!

"I'm gonna tell!" Mark threatened. I was scared to death. I had never held hands with a boy before. I was in unfamiliar territory and unsure of the degree of punishment that would entail. I was sure it would be bad, though. True to his word, as soon as we got home that night, Mark took great pleasure in telling on me. I held my breath in fear of what Daddy would say. To my shock and amazement, Daddy laughed. Mark was disappointed. I was relieved. Therefore, the next Friday night, I kissed Jimmy. Mark didn't see that.

I want to fast-forward about fifteen years now. The year was 1980. I was married, twenty-five, the mother of two boys—four and an infant. I had a very active social life as a "stay-at-home mom, interacting with other stay-at-home moms. This is when I met Maggie.

Maggie is Scottish, married to Dave, who is British, and they had two children, both girls, ages three and seven. Dave was an engineer working in Sandersville on a four-year contract with a British owned kaolin company. Maggie and I were both part of the social network of stay-at-home moms. We became good and lasting friends. Despite the fact that we have each moved around the country over the years, in opposite directions, we have

106

managed to stay in touch with each other—a couple of visits when Maggie lived in Texas and then in Alabama, where she currently resides, and a yearly phone call. Occasionally, we exchange Christmas cards.

Fast forward again to 1991. My diagnosis with Parkinson's disease was four years prior, but symptoms had been present for the past six years. I was working as Director of Social Services at a hospital 30 miles away in Milledgeville, Georgia. The stress associated with my job had caused my disease to progress to the point that I had to quit and find a less stressful job that didn't require commuting.

I went to work at one of the local nursing homes as social worker and activities director. It was here that I met and fell in love with Miss Emmeline, Jimmy's grandmother! I lost my beloved grandmother at sixteen. Miss Emmeline was the first person that I had ever met since my own grandmother's death that even came close to reminding me of Grandma. Miss Emmeline was a joy to know, and I loved her. I mourned her death just two years after meeting her.

Finally, I was caught up with living my life as a newly wed (when I remarried in 2000 after being divorced for fifteen years) and discovered that it had been at least three years since I had talked with Maggie.

July 7, 2005, Iraqi terrorists bombed four different train stations in London simultaneously. I sat watching the news, horrified, and immediately thought of Maggie. I knew that almost every year, Maggie would go to England for a month to six weeks. Where was she? I wondered. Where were Anna and Helen, Maggie's daughters, who would be twenty-eight and thirty-three by this time? I was trying to remember the last conversation I'd had with Maggie. Did she tell me Anna was living in England? A telephone call to her was long overdue.

I called Maggie. The person who answered the telephone was definitely Maggie. I definitely recognized that sleepy sounding Scottish accent with a hint of a southern drawl thrown in (I was great at calling early in the morning and waking her up). This was a voice of Maggie that I had never heard before, though.

"Hey, Maggie, it's Terrie."

"Oh, Terrie," she said, in a vague, far away sounding voice. This was not Maggie as I remembered her.

"I am calling to be sure you're all okay."

There was silence on her end. Again, "Maggie, this is Terrie, are ya'll okay?"

Another short silence followed by a dreamlike, "Yes, I'm okay."

I was really becoming concerned now. This conversation was not going like any conversation I had ever had with Maggie. Something was wrong. I knew it but couldn't figure out what. Did Maggie have Alzheimer's disease?

"Maggie, do you know who this is?"

"Yes, it's Terrie."

"What's wrong, Maggie?" I was very concerned now.

There was a long pause before Maggie finally responded in a very faint yet controlled voice. "Terrie, I'm going to have to get back in touch with you. I need to think about this for a bit. Give me your number, and I promise to call you soon." With that said, she hung up.

Baffled and alarmed, I started frantically trying to remember where Dave now worked. I needed to call him and find out what was wrong. Had they gotten a divorce? So many questions and possible scenarios popped into my mind. Every scenario one could imagine except for the correct one—the most horrible one imaginable.

While searching for Dave's number, my telephone rang. It was Dave calling me!

"Hi, Terrie, it's Dave here. Maggie just rang me and said that you had called her asking about everyone. She is going through a pretty hard time right now and asked me to call you and explain because she just can't do it right now."

"What in the world has happened, Dave? Maggie sounded terrible!"

"You apparently don't know," Dave responded, "but we lost Anna a year ago. She died of liver disease. Today is the anniversary of the day we buried her."

My heart felt like it was breaking. I didn't know!

July 16, 2005, I was reading the Sandersville Progress. There was an article about Jimmy. He was in London the day of the bombs, taking a course at a nearby University. He had been to one of the train stations that was bombed on many occasions. He very well could have been there on July 7 at the precise time of the bombing.

Anna had been dead for an entire year, and I didn't know it because I put off calling Maggie for three years. I know there's nothing I could have done for Anna. If I had called sooner, though, could I have done something for Maggie? What if?

Jimmy asks about me every time he sees my dad. I have never told him how much that means to me. I have never told him how much I loved his grandmother, Miss Emmeline. It could have been him at the train station July 7. What if?

I did two things that day. First, I called Maggie again. We laughed, I cried, we reminisced for an hour. Then I emailed Jimmy. I told him how much it meant to me for him to ask about me regularly. I also told him how much I loved Miss Emmeline.

P.S. It's been about a year since I wrote this piece. Since then, my own mother entered the same nursing home in which Miss Emmeline had stayed. Guess what room she is in? Room 219— Miss Emmeline's room!

# IT AIN'T NOTHING BUT A THANG

Johnny and I had exactly seven weeks from the time we met until our wedding day in which to form our philosophy on marriage. We were both still a little bruised from previous marriages and had vivid memories of all the things that didn't work in a marriage. We both had children from our previous marriage. He had three and I had two. We made a solemn promise long before our wedding day that no matter what, our children would ALWAYS come first. We agreed to disagree, when necessary, regarding our approaches toward parenting but always to be supportive of each other's decisions. That promise has proven many times through our marriage to be the number one promise that has gotten us through some potentially rough waters.

At forty-five and forty-three, we were starting our lives over as teenagers. In other words, we were poor. We lived in Johnny's childhood home for the first six months, with a for sale sign in the front yard. A potential buyer forced us to find another place to live quickly. With little time and even less money, we creatively financed probably the most sensible deal of either of our lives. We found a 1960s vintage mobile home sitting on an acre of land, complete with century old oak trees and a long neglected spring-filled pond. It could be ours for $20,000. We were so poor that we couldn't even scrape together that amount of money. We put together a creative seven-year owner-financing package and moved in within 30 days. Our monthly mortgage payment was a whopping $254.41.

Fortunately, both of us can see beauty in the beast. The interior of our newly acquired palace left everything to one's imagination. There was no carpet on the floor, no bathtub in the

111

bathroom, no kitchen sink, and no stove or refrigerator. We definitely had an immediate challenge. The first six months made for some creative living, to put it mildly. We moved in, July, 2000. During the first six months, John installed the bathtub, and we camped out with a primitive kitchen using an apartment size refrigerator, a microwave, a toaster oven, and an electric frying pan. I washed the dishes in the bathtub. In August, I underwent brain surgery for the second time; this time to insert a pacemaker-like stimulator in my brain.

At the same time I was in the operating room, John was in the waiting room going through DT's. He had previously had a bad intestinal virus and, after recovering from that, he decided to quit drinking. He made the decision, unbeknownst to me, that, if I could undergo brain surgery to improve the quality of our lives that he could contribute by giving up alcohol. He'll tell you that he is not an alcoholic because he doesn't go to meetings. He's just a retired drunk. It was more than a week later before I realized the sacrifice that he had made.

We spent Thanksgiving, 2000, back at Emory with another round of brain surgery, this one unplanned. The wires connecting my stimulator had broken, and I had to go back and be rewired.

The Sunday after Thanksgiving, John was driving me home trying to maneuver the car as carefully as he could in horrendous post-Thanksgiving traffic. I was looking like an alien from out of space with my partially shaved head and a row of staples across the top of my bald head, which looked like a railroad track.

John is a bit hard of hearing and when I'm a little "off," my speech is quite low in volume and my movements are in slow motion. I was curled up in a fetal position with my back to John so that I wouldn't stress out at his maniacal driving. I had to go to the bathroom. Watching the road signs, when we came up on a sign for the next rest area, I poked John on the leg, pointed to the sign, and softly mouthed the words, "Rest area."

John incorrectly interpreted what I said, thinking that I was doped up and was pointing to something out of the window and calling it wisteria. Knowing that wisteria was not in season, he humored me and said something about how nice that was as he drove right past the only rest area within seventy miles. My discomfort was growing with each mile and finally I saw a sign for a gas station and managed to yell, "Bathroom!" In a flash,

John realized what I was trying to tell him earlier so drove across three lanes of traffic at breakneck speed to the exit ramp and came to a screeching halt in front of the door of the gas station. He pulled me out of the car and we did the two-person shuffle, slow motion, into the gas station, past the wide-eyed attendant, and into the women's bathroom together. While I was slowly pulling my pants back up, John decided to take advantage of the opportunity and went to the bathroom, too. I was still too "off" to move out of the way in time. The backsplash from the toilet caused John to pee all over my leg. We started laughing as we shuffled back out the door past the stunned attendant, got in our car, and took off again, headed home. Once back in the car, John turned to me and said, "It ain't nothing but a thang, baby."

In a way, I guess that's been our motto in marriage and why it works for us. Most of the events that we go through in our daily lives "ain't nothing but a thang."

One day, not long after we married, I was feeling guilty about not contributing financially to our marriage. Jokingly, we agreed that we didn't marry the other one for our youth, our health, our good looks, or our money. After thinking about that for a few minutes, John amended that statement. Thinking about how poor we were when we married he said, "Hell, I did marry you for your money. You get a government check every month! That's about the only money we can count on having every month."

It ain't nothing but a thang!

# JUST CALL ME GRANDMA

There are definite advantages to being over fifty. One is the privilege of becoming a card-carrying member of AARP. With my membership, I receive a monthly magazine that has a nice crossword puzzle in it. I love crossword puzzles. If I go to Target's optical department to purchase my bi-focals, I can save 55%. I haven't actually tried that one to comment on it.

I happily discovered, recently, that because I'm over fifty and my husband is now fifty that my automobile insurance premiums went down. We have such a squeaky-clean driving record that, coupled with being fifty, if our premium goes down any lower, GEICO will soon be paying ME to have their insurance.

The number one advantage to being over fifty, for me, though, is becoming a Grandma. I know there is no set age for grandparenthood. My parents were 37 thirty-seven and forty when they became grandparents for the first time. My procreation and that of my sons', however, was a bit later getting started.

I have two sons—Matthew, 28, and David, 31. Neither shows any sign of settling down in a marriage in the next millennium. I was worried that I would have to resign myself to the role of being a terrific great-aunt to my sister's granddaughter. I took my role seriously and was very good at it, but I really was jealous of my sister.

But, duh! What was I thinking? I didn't just fall off the turnip truck yesterday. Even I know that one doesn't have to be married to have a baby. It sometimes is just an unplanned event. This unplanned event happened to Matthew. He seems to be attracted to girls with names like April, Melissa, and Tiffany who already have at least one child. Such was the case this time. He announced to me early on in his relationship with his current girlfriend, who, by the way, already has one young daughter, that she was pregnant and was sure that the baby was his. Despite much pleading and discussion, he refused to have a paternity test done. I knew that he had always wanted to have a child, so he had made up his mind that this would be his child despite any outside chance that it wasn't. (He did eventually have a paternity test done to prove that he is indeed the father.) Despite the pregnancy, it was an "on again – off again" relationship. I quit asking the status because it would change weekly. Matthew never wavered in his commitment to being the father of this "soon to be arriving baby." The due date was around my birthday, the end of October 2005.

Matthew was at my house October 13th. We were sitting outside under the oak tree by the pond discussing his girlfriend and her doctor's appointment that day. She told Matthew that she would call him after the appointment and give him the doctor's report on her condition. He received a phone call about noon from her. She was crying so hard that Matthew could not understand what she was saying. All he could decipher was that she was in the hospital. He hung up, ran towards his truck, calling out, over his shoulder, "I'll call you as soon as I know what's going on."

I paced the floor, holding the portable phone in my hand for over an hour before the phone call came. "I have a son," Matthew said, in an oddly strained voice.

"Is everything okay?" I asked.

"The baby is fine," he assured me. "He was born last night." I knew that the plans were for Matthew to accompany his girlfriend to the hospital and be present in the delivery room when the baby was born. Something had obviously happened to change that.

"Come to the hospital now, Mama. I can't talk right now but will explain it to you when you get here."

In a daze, I drove to Lexington, 25 miles from home, to the hospital where my grandson had been born. Matthew met me at the door of the room with a grim look on his face. I looked in the room and saw the baby's mother, her two-year-old daughter, and an unfamiliar male who I quickly found out was her long-time boyfriend and the father of her daughter. My grandson was lying in a crib on the other side of the room away from them. As I walked in the room, everyone silently walked out of the room, leaving Matthew and me in the room with my new grandson. I was baffled, confused, dazed, speechless, and thrilled, all at the same time. I picked my grandson up and sat in the rocking chair, rocking him—crying and staring at his little face and hands in awe. Matthew stayed in the room with me but neither of us spoke. We just sat and looked at the baby.

About thirty minutes had passed when the entourage came back into the room. I silently stood up, handed the baby to Matthew and walked out of the room. The mother never made eye contact with me.

I was at the end of the corridor when I heard, "Wait up, Mom. I will walk you out." Matthew was furious and confused. He had no more clue as to what was going to happen beyond the present moment. His future had just come and gone in a flash. He was still trying to process the fact that he, his girlfriend, and the baby would not be going home from the hospital to live happily ever after in a little white house with the picket fence.

We were no more than halfway down the front steps of the hospital when Matthew's cell phone rang. It was Matthew's girlfriend calling to tell him that she did not want the baby. "You can take him home with you tomorrow. The nurse is here with his birth certificate. What do you want to name him? Matthew sat down on the hospital steps with a stunned look on his face. Looking at him, I sat down, too.

"David Aubin Whitling" he said. A couple of minutes later, he hung up, turned to me with tears in his eyes, his voice cracking, and said, "I'm taking my son home with me tomorrow."

There are few times in my life when I am rendered speechless. This was one of them though. Hell, I was still getting used to the idea that I was actually a grandma now and that it was not just a dream. My mind was going in a thousand directions. There was so much to do to get ready for a newborn baby and less than 24 hours to get it done. Matthew and baby David would be coming home to my house. They would stay there until there was a better plan. The only thing I was certain of was that Matthew would be a terrific father (and mother).

Sitting on the hospital steps, still somewhat dazed by the rapidly changing turn of events, cell phones in hand, we each started networking with friends and family to gather necessary items needed to care for a newborn baby.

My first SOS telephone call was to my ex-husband's wife, Karen, of all people! Oddly, I immediately thought of her because I knew they were already on their fourth grandchild and she could easily gather the necessary equipment for us. In addition, I knew she could keep my ex-husband calm and rational. My second phone call was to my sister-in-law, Julie, the networking expert of the South. True to their word, within three hours, they were all on my doorstep heavily laden with infant car seat, bottles, formula, diapers, and the promise of tomorrow's delivery of a baby bed.

The first few weeks, frankly, were a weary fog. I was using muscles I hadn't used since Matthew had been a baby. Nevertheless, I was madly, head over heels in love with my first grandchild, David Aubin Whitling. I knew, as intense as that feeling was, that over time, it would grow stronger.

I'M FINALLY A GRANDMA! What an incredible feeling. It came easy for me to want to be a good grandma. I had the best model of my own—Grandma Dorman. I pray that I have the opportunity to be the same kind of grandma to David as Beatrice Florence was to me—a relationship that lasts beyond a lifetime.

The other day, David was lying across my legs as I rocked him and talked to a friend on the telephone. Fifteen minutes later, after much rocking and soft chatter, I looked down at David and saw that he was sleeping, peacefully and soundly. I immediately flashed back to my own childhood with Grandma Dorman. While she sat on the back porch and gossiped with her neighbors, I would lie across her legs as she scratched my back in rhythm with her talking. The low drone of the conversation would lull me into a peaceful, warm, and secure sleep.

Watch over us, Grandma and help me be the best Grandma I can be— just like you!

# *THE WAY IT IS*

One Pallidotomy and four Deep Brain Stimulation procedures—over 15 years—and guess what? I still have Parkinson's disease. More importantly, I'm still here. I'm wired from my collarbone to the depths of my brain and have battery packs implanted over each breast (and no, it didn't make my breasts look bigger). I go to my programmer ever three months, much like the Bionic Woman, to be fine-tuned. My bald head looks like a topographical map.

If I had known 15-20 years ago what I know today about the devastating impact Parkinson's disease would bring to my life, as well as to the lives of all those whom I love, I don't think I would have hung around to experience it or to put them through the turmoil. God, in his infinite wisdom, knows just how much a person can handle. When you are trying your best just to live your life one day at a time, before you realize it, it's been 25 years. I am still here, still riding the roller coaster that is part of the package deal when it's Parkinson's disease. I have spent 25 years determined that I would not be defeated by this bitch of a disease and, so far, I am winning.

Many days it doesn't feel like I am winning. Many days it feels like all the brain surgeries and all the medications are useless. This is the part of the roller coaster ride that I hate with a vengeance. These are what I call my Parkinson Moments. They can last from three to seven days without relief. These are the times I retreat from the world out of necessity, take my phone off the hook, have panic attacks, depression, uncontrollable crying and fear— fear that I am never going to feel normal again. I feel like a prisoner trapped in my own body, not knowing when or if I will be released. My speech is all but unintelligible, my cognitive

119

ability slows down, and the ability to think of the words I want to say are gone.

During these days of agony for me, I would suspect that John is going through a form of agony himself. Although I cannot speak for him, I know he is confronted with an impossibly inconsolable wife. He feels helpless because he can't fix it. He is a mechanic by profession and when a car has a problem, he can fix it and make it well. Life is different living with me. There is nothing he can do to ease the burden of the disease for either of us. Communication between the two of us is possible only because we know each other so well that I am able to simplify conversation with one or two key words. During my more functional days, John will tell me that I am a control freak and try to micro-manage everything and everybody. I don't deny it. What is interesting is that during these cycles, I become obsessed with not being able to move as I would like to, so I try to force movement, knowing it is only going to upset me even more.

I can hear John saying, "This is going to pass; it always does." Patience is not a virtue of mine. After twenty-five years of this, I still panic. I obsess over the possibility that the immobility is NEVER GOING AWAY. Thank God, that John is my voice of reason. Don't ever believe that the spouse does not have the disease, too. John also lives with it every single day of his life. There is no vacation for either of us.

# THE FUTURE

I have lost count of the number of times I have declared this book finished. For at least four years, I have truly thought that I had said all I had to say on the subject of Parkinson's disease and me. Without fail, something would happen that I felt I just HAD to put in this book.

I am fifty-three years old now. I have been writing this book for over ten years. A lot has happened in those ten years. I have lost several very good friends to their battles with Parkinson's disease. Steve Mulligan was the first, in 1997. Millie Kondracke was next. Many of you have read the book that her husband, Mort, wrote about her. There was also my Baptist Preacher friend, John Cann, and my New York friend, Bill Thorson. Last but certainly not least was my very dear friend George Rollin (Rol) Parker III. The question keeps coming to me, "Why them and not me?" I have battled the same disease for as long as they have, longer than some. Yet I am still here living, loving, and battling this monster daily. I said in the beginning of this book that I felt like God allowed me the opportunity to live with this disease for a very specific reason. Over the years, I think the reasons have changed, but I still think I am here, living with Parkinson's, for a reason. Because I feel strongly about this, I feel that my responsibility is to do all that is within my power to live with this disease as independently as I possibly can. This means to take advantage of all available forms of treatment that are appropriate for me at this time.

I underwent a Pallidotomy in 1993, when the medical professionals considered it a very new and somewhat experimental procedure. Later, in 2000, shortly after my marriage to John, I underwent Deep Brain Stimulation to improve my functional level. Seven years later, now, and I have just undergone Bilateral Deep Brain Stimulation. It is important to me that I function at a higher level than I am now. I find myself growing more dependent on others for help.

I have people that need me, though: my husband, John, needs me so that he does not have to face life alone. My grandson, David, needs a Grandma (me), one who is active, capable, competent, and fun. I have barely begun to give him the kind of relationship that Grandma gave to me. I know that this gift will be with him forever in his heart. Gail needs me because I will be her strength when our parents die. My son, David, needs me. I have always been his best cheerleader, and he still needs one. He has embarked on a new and exciting career, at thirty-one, and needs the excitement and enthusiasm that I have always had for whatever new challenge he undertakes. Matthew needs me. He knows that out of everybody in his world, I am the ONE person that he always knows he can count on. Daddy needs me. It would literally break his heart to lose another child during his lifetime. I know there are countless others that need me, too; others with Parkinson's disease, who, by my example, will challenge themselves to live with their disease with dignity and courage.

This is where I choose to end this book. Why now, you might be wondering, when the outcome of my treatment is unknown? My life has been about independence, courage, fearlessness, and confidence. I know that I will be better. There is no doubt in my mind that Bilateral Deep Brain Stimulation will restore my functional level to that which will be acceptable to me for many years to come. Maybe I'll title my next book, *The Bionic Grandma.*

I believe
that everything
happens for a reason—
even this!
Jennie